Women on Hysterectomy *or* How long before I can hang-glide?

by

Nikki Henriques & Anne Dickson

Cover illustrations by Kate Charlesworth

THORSONS PUBLISHING GROUP LIMITED
Wellingborough * New York

First published 1986

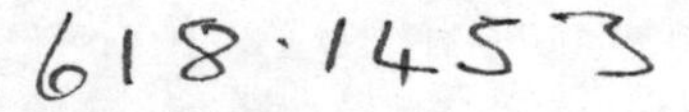

British Library Cataloguing in Publication Data

Henriques, Nikki
Women on hysterectomy : how long before I can hang glide?—(whole woman books)
1. Hysterectomy
I. Title II. Dickson, Anne III. Series
618.1'453 RG391

ISBN 0-7225-1164-7

Printed and bound in Great Britain

Contents

DEDICATION

This book is written in celebration of women's remarkable powers of physical and emotional endurance.

Foreword

The number of women who each year lose their uterus, and sometimes with it the ovaries, is very, very large.

The operation may be done for any one of a number of reasons, ranging from the obviously essential need to rid a woman of a cancerous growth, to dealing with period problems that are due as much (if not more) to emotional disease as to physical disease.

It may even be done, in a few cases, because it is in a sense a 'fashionable' operation. We aren't quite as likely to have that happen here in Britain as it used to be in America, where many women have been unnecessarily stripped of their uteruses (and many surgeons' pockets made agreeably plump in consequence) since the British National Health Service tends to block that sort of bad medicine.

But all the same, there are women who go through this major surgical experience with little or no prior discussion of what it might mean to them, or why it actually needs to be done, and who get scant help afterwards. I know because they write me letters in their hundreds, asking for that sort of help and information.

So I welcome this book wholeheartedly. It's about as close as a woman can get to sitting round a comfortable kitchen table with her elbows propped up over a cup of coffee, talking to other women who've had the experience. That sort of information and support garnering can be the best there is, as any self-help group can tell you.

And in a sense, the book is better than a casually constituted group of talking women, because it can happen that such a group will include one or two who have totally erroneous information to impart, or who are motivated by an unpleasant wish to frighten and shock. And yes, there are women like that, though happily there are fewer of them than some critics of women's groups would lead you to believe.

Certainly there is nothing in these pages that will frighten or shock you gratuitously. Neither, however, is there any sort of whitewash job. Doctors and nurses will sometimes say, well meaningly, 'Oh, it's nothing – you'll be fine in two ticks – soon be all better!' and that makes a woman who needs rather longer than two ticks to get back on her feet feel ashamed and guilty. What such a woman needs – what *all* women need – is honest information, honestly given.

And this book provides just that, on a subject that concerns many women. It really is a pleasure to welcome it to the armoury of women's information banks.

CLAIRE RAYNER

Introduction

This book came into being as a direct result of Nikki's hysterectomy. Although her experience was positive, she was astonished at her own lack of knowledge of her body and the general lack of information about the operation and its aftermath.

This book is a product of our joint words, thoughts and skills.

Our intention has been to provide a book which will be of interest to women who have already had a hysterectomy and to women who are contemplating the operation; to their families and friends and to their GPs, nurses and surgeons, who as a result of reading what women say themselves may be better equipped to inform their patients appropriately and to offer the best possible support and care.

We would like to acknowledge our debt to the following people:

All the women who agreed to be interviewed about their experience – Jo, Christine, Jane, Francesca, Ann, Linda, Maureen, Sheila, Sue, Claire, Erica, Elisabeth, and Sonia who provided us with the rich and illuminating material on which we have based our book.*

The consultant gynaecologist to whom Nikki has reason to be personally thankful for the successful outcome of her operation, but to whom we both wish to express very sincere thanks for his time in being interviewed on several occasions and for agreeing to act in a consultative capacity for this book, as well as giving us a lot of support and encouragement along the way. We are not able to name him for the usual ethical reasons but we hope his generosity to us will in some measure be rewarded by our providing an

*We have changed the names of the women interviewed in the text to retain confidentiality.

anonymous platform for some of his deeply-felt convictions! The Women's Health Information Centre, the BMA Press Office for the use of their facilities.

Special thanks to Claire Rayner for agreeing to write the foreword, and for her help.

To Gillian Wadsted who acted as chief scout, informing us of relevant articles and programmes; Deirdre Sanders, Sonia Bull, Jean Hopwood, Chris Christophe and Judy Vaughan of the Hysterectomy Support Group, all of whom put us in touch with interviewees.

To the Staff Nurse and Dr Elphis Christopher who took time out of their very busy lives to talk to us and share their views.

We have been very impressed and moved by what these women have had to say and we treasure the experience. Nearly all our interviewees told us that the interview provided them with the first real opportunity to talk in depth about their views, their feelings and their experience of their hysterectomy. There must be many more women who have never spoken, and no doubt there will be many more in the future.

We hope that this book will encourage those women to break the silence.

NIKKI HENRIQUES AND ANNE DICKSON

1

Fear of the Unknown

Although the experience of hysterectomy wasn't greatly influenced by general myths among the women interviewed, nonetheless we found that there were very real individual fears.

Some of these fears related to the experience of having any major operation. 'Most women are frightened of the operation itself, and the anaesthetic. Very frightened because they think they will not wake up.' (*Staff Nurse*)

Our consultant, too, said one of the most pressing worries for patients was whether they were going to die.

Jenny was 'frightened of the anaesthetic', and Jean was similarly 'terrified'. Angela resisted the advice she was given to have a hysterectomy for two years, because 'my experience of operations and anaesthetics has never been a very happy one. I thought, one of these days I'll go under . . . .' Apart from her fear of not coming round afterwards, her reluctance was strengthened by unpleasant reactions to the anaesthetic. This same adverse reaction was described by Jean and Louise.

In view of these fears, Staff Nurse felt the anaesthetist was a very good person to talk to patients. In her hospital they usually saw the anaesthetist before the operation, so patients knew who was going to administer the anaesthetic. 'They recognize their face in theatre, which is reassuring.' (*Staff Nurse*)

Cancer

Also preying on the minds of many women was the fear of cancer.

'If you have a gynaecological symptom, depending on your age, all sorts of anxieties present themselves: if you're young, you're worried that you will never be able to have children. And if you have had children, then you are worried that this might be the first sign of cancer.' (*Gynae*)

Staff Nurse mentioned this same fear: 'They think the word *fibroids** is cancerous as well. That's a word they don't understand. It's very important that we explain it and as soon as the results come back, to show them written evidence that there is no sign of cancer.'

Jean had been informed that she had a patch on her cervix which could have been cancerous. For her in particular the possibility of cancer profoundly affected her whole experience of hysterectomy, and influenced her decision not to confide in her husband because she didn't want to alarm him.

Margaret was admitted to hospital and after all the preliminary tests, was suddenly asked to go home, because 'they had a girl who had gone to the clinic that day and they wanted to operate immediately . . . that girl had cancer and that was it. So that relieved my mind, because if they had thought the same about me, I would have been done that day.'

Carole's fears grew over the period of time (seven months) she had to wait to have her operation. 'The longer I had to wait, the more it played on my mind. I worried. Why did I have to have the operation? What were they going to find? Was it cancer, like everybody said? What was the reason for it? I tried to put it to the back of my mind and just couldn't. What about complications? When I get frightened, I get the runs. So the last week I was for ever in the toilet.'

The same fear contributed to Louise's decision to go ahead: 'I felt it had to be done because I could have had cancer. It was a mess in there.'

Another real fear is how long one is going to be an invalid after the operation.

Lack of mobility

Jean: 'I was worried about not being able to cope. How weak will I be? Other people are three months unable to do anything. Or is it three months? Is it just the two weeks in hospital that I'm going to feel weak? How will the children get to school?'

She also expressed anxiety about losing her independence: 'Being totally dependent – that was my real fear.' Jenny shared this: 'I was frightened of how long it would be before I could be

*For definitions of all clinical terms, see Glossary on page 139.

mobile, and not tied to tubes, be independent again.'

The gynaecologist agreed this was a common concern: 'How soon are they going to recover; when are they going to be able to do the things they had been told they might not be able to do?' All these fears are understandable and could be much better coped with if more information were easily available and women were encouraged to ask more questions. Fear is compounded by an inadequate knowledge of our own bodies.

A need for information

Even though we found each woman's experience of hysterectomy was different, the universal theme encountered was the importance of information and the high level of anxiety engendered by the lack of it.

This applied even to those women who had received some medical training: 'Just because I was a nurse it didn't mean I knew everything that was going on. I did my gynae nursing years ago – so why should I know what was going to happen? (*Sandra*)

Much of our difficulty is inevitably a result of not knowing how our body works; this applies in general to the bowel, lungs, kidneys, blood circulation, and in particular to the reproductive system. As the gynaecologist said: 'We haven't been taught enough about how our bodies work . . . there are lots of opportunities in a woman's life where she should be taught about the function of the womb and genital tract, but for various reasons that doesn't take place.'

This lack of education leads to fundamental ignorance about our anatomy and is why many women do not understand what happens in hysterectomy.

Louise: 'I wasn't told whether they would just take the uterus or the ovaries as well, tubes or what they were taking. I didn't know. I must admit I thought there was a great big hole because no one told me any different. I thought they had taken half my insides away and that I was left with a gap. I couldn't understand how I did have a gap, or where or what the remaining bits were.'

'In the convalescent home there were so many women there who had the operation but didn't know what had been taken out.' (*Sally*)

'Is there a hole inside? Do they neaten it off? What happens if you have a womb and they cut it off? How do they treat it? Do they stitch that bit up or what? It's still a question in my mind.' (*Margaret*)

Staff Nurse: 'They think they are going to be completely stitched up, especially if they are going to have a vaginal hysterectomy . . . that word vagina. They don't realize they won't have periods any more as they don't have a uterus. They ask if they will get pregnant.'

One of the worst consequences of ignorance is that we are frightened about what is going to happen and often too anxious or embarrassed to enquire.

Staff Nurse: '[They are] very, very nervous on admission for the simple reason they don't know anything and they are too frightened to ask.'

'I felt a fool not knowing my own body. I felt quite ashamed of myself really.' (*Jean*) She was fortunate and found someone sympathetic and prepared to take the time to answer her questions. 'Dr B's registrar came round and I said "You might think I'm daft, but there are a couple of things I just don't know. What's going to be at the top? If you take everything away is it going to be open? Closed? Shorter or longer?" Her response was to roar with laughter in a very nice way and say: "Goodness me, let me draw you a diagram." She drew me a square indicating the vagina and said, "We sew along the top and leave the rest intact." I thought well, that's good, because that worried me. I had thought perhaps they just neaten it off and you are left with this vacuum and all your innards exposed.'

All the women we interviewed were asked whether they felt they had sufficient information before the operation, or whether they would have liked more. In general, their answers conveyed a wish for more information about the operation itself, about the hospital and about recovery.

'I wasn't told what would happen in the operation or anything at all. I was seven months on the waiting list. On admission another doctor examined me and said, "You'll have it done tomorrow morning; you'll go through your change when you are fifty," and that was all I was told. There was no one to discuss it with. How I was going to wake up, what medication I'd be on. There were no other patients to talk things over with.' (*Carole*)

'They didn't really give me much information about hysterectomy. I think they took it for granted that because I had had a previous operation to remove an ovary, I would know.' (*Sally*)

'I wanted to read in what way I would be weakened, whether it would be painful or ache. I would like to have known how other people related to it.' (*Jean*)

Whose responsibility is it to inform patients of what is about to happen to them and why? 'When patients are admitted, I would like to think that a young doctor would sit with the sister on the gynae ward and they could talk with the patient for forty minutes about hysterectomy. The sister on the gynae ward is the best person. The most important thing in looking after patients is talking to them.' (*Gynae*)

'I think it's our job, or better still the doctor should tell them what to expect before they even come to the ward. When they come in we try and explain what they are going to have done, but this is really the doctor's job.' (*Staff Nurse*)

Is it the consultant's job or should it be the GP – the first person patients are likely to contact about their symptoms? Or should it be the nurse; or need it be a person at all, why not something to read?

'I would like to see a booklet handed out to every patient as soon as they know they are to be admitted. They can read up on it and start asking questions when they come in . . . We can then put their minds at rest.' (*Staff Nurse*)

We discovered that literature does exist in some hospitals. Sally had a 'very good booklet' given to her when she was admitted to hospital but not before. But this is far from common practice: it's usually left to the initiative of the patient to find out what she can from whoever she can. 'My husband went out and bought me a book on hysterectomy and I sat down and read it all.' (*Carole*)

'I went through all the books in the library, every article I could lay my hands on.' (*Sally*)

'The only information I had at the time was given to me by a friend who had the operation six years before, and she had a photocopy of an old BMJ article on hysterectomy which told me virtually nothing.' (*Jean*)

'I knew a bit about it because a friend of mine in Bristol had had one a long time ago. I knew they took the womb away and that it was like any other operation.' (*Fiona*)

If there is one thing that can be said to be a common denominator among our interviewees it was that as women we are very ignorant about our bodies and that information *helps*. However, in deciding who is responsible for providing information, we need to take into account two very human factors. First, not everyone wants to know the same things. In fact, some people claim to be happier remaining totally ignorant. Second, we need to be told things more than once before they can be fully absorbed.

The essence of imparting information clearly can be summed up in terms of *correct timing* and *reinforcement*. Whatever we are told in advance about recovery for example, it is only when you struggle to get out of bed or wonder how soon you can drive the car, that the relevant information has any meaning.

Our ability to retain the information and advice is affected by the anxiety and vulnerability of being a patient and dependent on strangers for survival. Given the distressing circumstances, it would seem that all medical personnel, GPs, consultant and nursing staff, should be sensitive and open to patients' need for information, regardless of how trivial it may seem to them, or how often it has been asked before. As our Staff Nurse said: 'The questions might seem silly, but they are very important to the patient . . . I don't think we can talk to patients enough.'

A common argument against giving information to patients is: 'They say if we tell you too much, you'll forget or it may not happen to you.' (*Sally*) But this negative attitude gives no credit to the patient's commonsense. Every woman we interviewed took it for granted that the experience of the operation and recovery would be different for each woman, and would depend on a particular combination of individual factors. Nevertheless they wanted more information, and medical practitioners who withhold information on the grounds that it may not happen, would appear to do most of their patients a gross disservice.

Some of the women reported they had received all the information they required. Celia and Fiona and Jenny said their consultants had given them all the information they requested but Jenny added, 'I was just like anyone else leaving the discussion, not being able to remember what I had been told.' Their statements referred to information received before the operation.

Another area of concern was wanting information *after* the operation: what had been found and what had been removed. Angela was fortunate: 'They were very good about coming immediately after the operation, to tell you what they had done and how everything was. I felt that was very good.'

But on the whole, that type of information is not made available to the patient, even though such a request is quite reasonable.

Information on what has been lost or found, is especially important in view of the real fears about cancer. Even in situations when cancer had not been specifically mentioned as a possibility, there is still a secret fear that prompts the need for unmistakeable evidence to the contrary.

From our interviews the two areas adequately covered were recovery and sexual activity. This information was given by doctors, nurses or consultants although the amount and content varied considerably. (These areas are covered more fully in Chapters 8 and 10.) It would appear that requests for information on sexual intercourse and recovery are expected by the medical profession, whereas requests for information about our anatomy and physiology and the physical and emotional readjustments are seldom anticipated. Perhaps it's because it takes more time but surely such information can help. As our gynaecologist said: 'An understanding of what has happened is one of the factors which contribute to a more rapid recovery.'

2
Hearing the News

An important element in the experience of being in hospital and recovery from surgery is a woman's reaction to having a hysterectomy in the first place – whether she welcomes it as a relief or whether it represents an unwanted solution.

Positive choice or an unwelcome necessity?

'For me it was a positive choice to have a hysterectomy. Finding a gynaecologist who took me seriously and who agreed to hysterectomy was a tremendous relief.' (*Nikki*)

Several of the women interviewed regarded hysterectomy as a positive choice. After years of troublesome periods Elaine 'asked for hysterectomy although there was no reason medically why I should have one . . . I had three children and thought I would try and get rid of the thing.'

Sandra had a similar experience: 'I wanted a hysterectomy because it was a drain every month and it was getting costly. I was more than happy to have it out.' Fiona too was 'very pleased. It was what I had been trying for all those years.'

Margaret welcomed the news because her periods had long been a nuisance to her: 'I was glad to get rid of it. It has given me so much pain. I had three children and I certainly didn't want any more.' She was so delighted that she described hysterectomy as 'The best thing since marmalade!'

Celia was motivated to have a hysterectomy by the continual pain of sexual intercourse. 'It didn't bother me that I was going to have it. My husband had a vasectomy eight years before, so we didn't want any more children anyway.' If a woman has taken a clear decision that she doesn't want more children, it can be easier to accept the idea of hysterectomy.

It seems that even if a woman has decided not to have more children, her reaction can still be one of shock, simply because we tend to associate hysterectomy with a woman who is older and at the end of her reproductive cycle. 'At first I was a bit shocked: I wasn't sure I wanted to take that step. I was only twenty-nine when it was suggested.' For this reason Sally held out for a while. 'I kept thinking maybe it will get better, something will happen in between.' She asked for time to consider hysterectomy and was told there was nothing else they could suggest. Nevertheless she decided first to try alternative treatment before making the final decision.

The surprised reaction of a younger woman having a hysterectomy can also be expressed by those around her: 'My friends were quite shocked. I think it was to do with my age [thirty-one]' Jenny also felt she couldn't discuss it for the same reason. 'No one at work had much idea of what was going on. I was ashamed of having a hysterectomy at the age of thirty.' But despite this she did think that a hysterectomy might solve her problems. She wanted very much to be physically fit again.

For Ellen the news was extremely upsetting, because it crystallized her personal conflict with her husband about the possibility of having another child: 'When the letter came telling me I had to go in, I went to pieces, cried and cried. I had to face the loss of my uterus, the possibility of not having any more children, and I didn't want to face it. I felt miserable and just cried. I rang my sister because I couldn't stop crying and she came straight over. She rang the surgery because she thought I was anaemic again – given to weeping. Talking it over with the doctor I realized it was just the shock of the letter. I had to go through with it. So I opted out of the responsibility. What I said to my GP was that I didn't actually want to stop having children. Really I wanted all along to have more children. I now had to face the knowledge that I wouldn't have any more.'

Louise opted for hysterectomy but wished she hadn't: 'I did want another child, I had been trying so long. By then my daughter was nine and I was still desperately trying for another one. And I knew if I had a hysterectomy that was it, it was finished, there's no going back. I think adjusting to the fact I couldn't have any more children was the worst.'

Anticipation

Your reaction to being told you are to have a hysterectomy will be influenced by whether or not you know what to expect.

'I was only thirty, one of the youngest in there. I didn't know anything. Oh God! I was petrified. I really was.' Louise had been given no information about the operation, therefore her worst fantasies consisted of memories of being in hospital before. 'Every time I had a miscarriage and went into hospital, I saw all these people having had hysterectomies and I thought, 'Oh God, that's something I never want to have.' I was so frightened when I saw them on these drips and the way they walked around afterwards. I thought *NO!*'

Fear of the unknown affected Jean's reaction in a different way. She saw hysterectomy as a positive solution; she had been told she might have cancer. 'I didn't worry about losing my womb to keep alive. I was far more worried about not being able to cope. I can remember coming back on the train. I gave myself to the end of the journey to come to terms with the fact that this was what was going to happen. I can remember sitting there blinking back tears. I was worried what I was going to do with the children.'

Time to think

'I believe it is important for patients to have time to come to terms with the decision.' (*Gynae*)

Sally gave herself plenty of time to think before making the final decision. 'Once I made the decision it was pretty easy. Once I had made up my mind, I don't think I had that many doubts; I saw it as the only way out.'

Having the time to think and talk through all the implications of hysterectomy is *crucial*. Sometimes this happens naturally if you have been suffering pain or distressing symptoms over a period of time. You can begin to look forward to the possibility of hysterectomy, or at least feel resigned to it, by the time the gynaecologist actually spells it out.

'I had worked out before going to see the surgeon that hysterectomy was what he was going to offer. I didn't want to keep having anaesthetics and repair jobs every three years. When I saw him it was hanging round my knees yet again. He said: "Right, we'll whip that out!" It wasn't a shock or a surprise.' (*Celia*)

However, it does not appear that time to think is considered a woman's right by all gynaecologists. It seems to be more a question of luck than right. Two of the women interviewed were very 'unlucky': Louise was referred to a gynaecologist for a private consultation. Having examined her, he announced: 'It's entirely up to you, but the state your stomach is in now, I would like to do a hysterectomy within two weeks.' He told Louise, 'The best thing to do is whip the whole lot out.' Anyway he didn't give her long to decide. 'He gave me half an hour, there and then in which to make up my mind.' Even though the prospect of not having any more children was for Louise very painful and traumatic, there was no sensitivity shown to her in this gynaecologist's approach.

Carole wasn't bothered by not having more children, but she too found the shock announcement very traumatic; especially so because of hearing the news while lying on her back, undergoing an internal vaginal examination: 'I was under the observation of a dozen strangers when I heard. I thought I would probably be going in for a scrape. But I heard the news in front of students, nurses and the consultant. They were really young men and women. I didn't know he was going to come out with the idea of hysterectomy. The words he used were "You need to have a hysterectomy. Do you want it or not?" That was it. I said "You're the doctor, you tell me. What can I say?" He said, "You'd be better off without it, sitting there doing nothing – it'll get rid of the pain and heavy periods." I said, "Yes, okay." He said, "Put your name on the list and you'll be hearing from us."'

Without ever being offered an alternative, or being told anything about what would happen in the operation, Carole then had to wait for seven months before going into hospital, getting more and more anxious as the time approached.

Carole's experience is a far cry from the approach advised and taught to medical students. 'The first question I ask before saying "You need a hysterectomy" – because it's a terrible shock – is: "What has your doctor told you?" If the patient hasn't been warned by her GP then I've got to be very sensitive. When I give people news of great emotional portent, bad news or the need for a serious operation, I try and talk to them so they think of what I'm going to say before I actually have to say it.

'I try and get them to think of it first. Many say, "You're not talking about hysterectomy are you?" Then they feel they have joined in the discussion and that this is the sensible and logical thing.' (*Gynae*)

If this sounds a little manipulative, it seems preferable to the hit and run approach suffered by Carole and Louise. Furthermore, this particular gynaecologist is sincerely open to the fact that a woman might not agree with his prognosis.

'Their response might be *"No"*. And I say: "Fine! But let's not settle for 'No' just yet. Go home and talk to your partner, family, your GP, any friends who have had the operation and come and see me again soon."' (*Gynae*)

To confront a woman with a shock announcement and to push her into the distressing situation of being forced to decide on such an important matter without giving her alternatives or information or time to reflect, can only be described as abusive. But apart from the brutality of it, it doesn't actually make sense. Anyone under such stress cannot think clearly or even *listen* clearly to what's being said.

'If you sit someone up and say, "Right, you've got to have a hysterectomy," and they hadn't thought they were going to have one, the emotional impact of that is so great, no matter what you say to them for the next three hours, they won't understand.' (*Gynae*)

Clearly the best way for a woman to assimilate information and make her own decision is to have enough time to think. And if this sort of announcement *has* to be made with others present as happens in teaching hospitals, then there are more sensitive ways of handling the situation.

Evidently, as we cannot always expect to be given the time to think, it is very important that we are able to ask for all the information we need in order to make this decision. (See Chapter 5.)

3
Why Hysterectomy?

Hysterectomy certainly counts as a common operation for women, but its incidence is not as high as is popularly assumed. Our gynaecologist placed it *fifth* on his list of common operations – termination of pregnancy, evacuation of a spontaneous miscarriage, 'D and C' and laparoscopy being more common. Nevertheless, approximately 1,000 hysterectomies are carried out, in Britain alone, each week.

Why is it done?

The most common symptom motivating women to seek help is excessive bleeding and pain caused by heavy irregular periods (Dysfunctional Uterine Bleeding).

'I had continual heavy periods lasting up to three weeks. It was difficult to say when one stopped and the next began.' (*Angela*)

'My GP put me on the pill to regularize my period but it didn't work – I was still flooding.' (*Margaret*)

'One day, while erecting an exhibition display, I realized I was dripping blood all over the marble floor. It really did come on quite suddenly about eighteen months before my operation. I had had a D and C about twelve months before, but was told I would need a hysterectomy at some time in the future.' (*Sandra*)

Louise suffered a long history of gynaecological problems: 'I had six miscarriages and one abortion at five months. I had very heavy periods, haemorrhaging and was always in and out of hospital.'

Ellen said: 'I had very heavy periods and was severely anaemic. I had a D and C and injections but it was just as bad after the D and C.'

Penny told us: 'I had a lot of trouble for two years. When I had intercourse it washed all over the floor.'

'I went to the doctor originally because I had three days each month when I didn't have a period. I had had a D and C after my youngest child (two years before). I just had non-stop bleeding. I started to get less and less time between periods and spotting in between. I had tremendous backache and was irritable and disorientated as well – I didn't notice pain having babies, but with this, I was taking nine Paracetamol every night in order to sleep. My skin was terrible, I was terribly tired and very run-down. It was as if I wasn't in my own body. As if I was watching someone else live my life. I was so tired, I'd have to lie down at the slightest thing and I'd be quite numb.' (*Jean*)

'I asked for a hysterectomy although there was no reason medically why I should have one. I found periods extremely annoying, inconvenient and generally tiresome. As I got older they got worse and heavier and I had several bad embarrassing anti-social accidents.' (*Elaine*)

'I had very heavy periods, pain in my side. Sex was really painful. I had these symptoms for eighteen months. The pain was so severe I couldn't even hoover.' (*Carole*) Seven years before she had undergone another operation to correct her tilted womb; she was sterilized at the same time.

Sally also suffered menstrual irregularities: 'I had ovulation pain, heavy periods and PMT. They weren't sure if it was all linked together. Two years before my hysterectomy I had an ovary removed but my complaint actually worsened after that.'

In order to understand the cause of excessive and irregular bleeding more clearly, we need to understand how the body functions normally.

A remarkable pattern

In the normal course of the menstrual cycle, the hormones oestrogen and progesterone are produced by the follicle (egg sac) which in turn produces a ripe egg each month: oestrogen as the egg ripens and develops, progesterone as the egg is released from the ovary.

Part of the ovary which develops as the egg develops is called the *corpus luteum*. This has a fixed life of fourteen days and part of its function is to produce progesterone.

The effect of maintaining the progesterone level is that the lining of the womb (the endometrium) thickens with the increased blood supply providing a plush environment in which to accommodate the fertilized egg. It waits for fourteen days for a successful union between egg and sperm but if that doesn't occur within that time, the corpus luteum gives up on its task, dies, disintegrates and is eventually absorbed into the body.

When this happens the effect is dramatic. The progesterone level suddenly falls. This affects a woman's body in terms of her moods, appetite, balance, mobility and the lining of the womb (endometrium) is particularly affected. The blood vessels which supply the endometrium go into spasm because of the lack of progesterone; their walls break and haemorraging occurs. The endometrium is shed in a very special and remarkable way. It comes away from the womb and what we know as our 'period' is over in about five days.

Irregular or prolonged bleeding

At either extreme of our reproductive life – as young girls starting to menstruate or women over thirty-five to forty, when we approach the time we are going to stop – the normal cycle can be upset when our ovaries do not produce eggs (ovulation).

If we do not ovulate the *corpus luteum* will not be produced, which means there will be no progesterone hormone. This in turn means there will be no normal shedding of the womb lining. When this happens the follicle (egg sac) which produces oestrogen disintegrates fairly quickly after fourteen days, or slowly after six weeks.

As it disintegrates the level of oestrogen falls slowly, and the womb lining (endometrium) is also shed, but not in the same way as in the normal cycle which regularly occurs due to the fall in progesterone. This time it is shed in response to the lack of oestrogen and it occurs in an irregular and prolonged way – heavy, irregular bleeding.

Women suffering in this way will often have no idea of when their period is due, and not know – when it does arrive – whether it will last a couple of days or three weeks; all very unpredictable.

When this upset in the ovulatory cycle occurs in teenage girls before their bodies settle down, treatment usually involves administration of hormones such as the contraceptive Pill, in anticipation of their pattern of menstruation taking over: their reproductive function lies ahead of them.

However, when it happens to a woman at the end of her reproductive phase as she becomes less fertile, the usual treatment is hysterectomy, because it is considered, 'It's all finished with'. Our consultant said: 'If we could give patients their premenstrual progesterone in the way they should take it, we'd reduce the number of hysterectomies.'

Sometimes patients are given added progesterone in tablet form, which must be taken five to ten days before their period is due. But there appear to be a number of difficulties with this kind of treatment caused according to the consultant, by women not understanding how their bodies work. The consequence of this confusion is that:

1. They don't take the treatment properly
2. They don't take it for long enough
3. They probably start too late
4. After three months they feel they can't take it any more and opt for hysterectomy.

Other reasons for hysterectomy are pelvic inflammatory disease (PID) and prolapsed womb.

'I had PID for a number of years which was probably connected to the fact I had a contraceptive coil fitted earlier, and I had an abortion some years earlier; and appendicitis. All of which caused lots of adhesions [lumps of fibrous tissue]. I had a number of laparoscopies and division of adhesions. I continued to have problems and my gynaecologist suggested I have a hysterectomy.' (*Jenny*)

'I had a repair job [re-stitching of prolapsed womb] three years before, which had gone wrong. We couldn't make love any more because it was so painful. I realized the repair job had fallen apart.' (*Celia*)

There are two more reasons for performing hysterectomy – the attitude expressed by some doctors of whipping it all out at once under the premise that women don't want more than one operation in their life, and they're better off without it anyway; and the decision taken by women to seek hysterectomy for particular symptoms even though no medical reason can be discovered.

What we know now about the menstrual cycle is not the whole

story – we've still got a lot to learn.

We know that menstruation is easily affected by stress: air hostesses constantly flying through time zones have period problems; women moving from one country to another may experience period problems; and 'The nicest thing you can say to a woman marrying between her periods is "Wear a Tampax" because as they walk up the aisle they'll start to bleed.' (*Gynae*) A stressful event such as bereavement can also cause women to bleed – sometimes this continues unabated.

We know also that menstruation often stops completely when we are emotionally disturbed, particularly when we are depressed. The link between our emotional state and our physical symptoms is often obvious yet difficult to pinpoint, because we don't know enough about the scientific mechanism. Living in a world where only scientific and rational explanation is acceptable, our observations and knowledge which come from our emotional and intuitive faculties are easily overlooked and dismissed.

But although it is difficult to determine exactly the emotional contribution to bodily symptoms, two of the women we interviewed said that although they were bleeding heavily, no physical cause was ever established.

It is possible that Ellen's experience was affected by the impasse in her relationship with her husband. She very much wanted another child, but he was adamant in his refusal. Her heavy bleeding coincided with her inability to find a solution to the situation.

Similarly, it is possible that Carole's severe abdominal pain in her right side and heavy bleeding was affected by the traumatic experience of a compulsory termination of pregnancy after her baby had died in her womb, combined with the insensitive treatment she received in hospital at the time. As she told us, 'When they analysed the womb the day after the operation, it was found to be perfectly healthy.' (*Carole*) No medical explanation was found for the very real suffering experienced by both women.

Jenny showed some insight into this link between body and feelings. Her husband had been married before and did not want any more children. Her conflict between the love for her husband and her wish to have children was unresolved. She said she felt that, in a way, her body 'complied' as the symptoms which erupted led to the need for her operation.

Excessive bleeding is a very common symptom from which women seek relief, the treatment of which may ultimately end in hysterectomy. So far we have considered how that happens when all the reproductive organs themselves are healthy, but the delicate mechanism which controls their function is faulty. The other common cause of excessive bleeding and menstrual disorders is when one or more of the organs has become diseased.

Fibroids

Fibroids are lumps of fibrous tissue which grow in the muscle of the womb (uterus). They can occur at any time during the reproductive phase of life, and are very common, but particularly so in women over forty. Fibroids are thought to be dependent on the hormone oestrogen for their growth because they often grow quickly during pregnancy when oestrogen levels are higher than at other times.

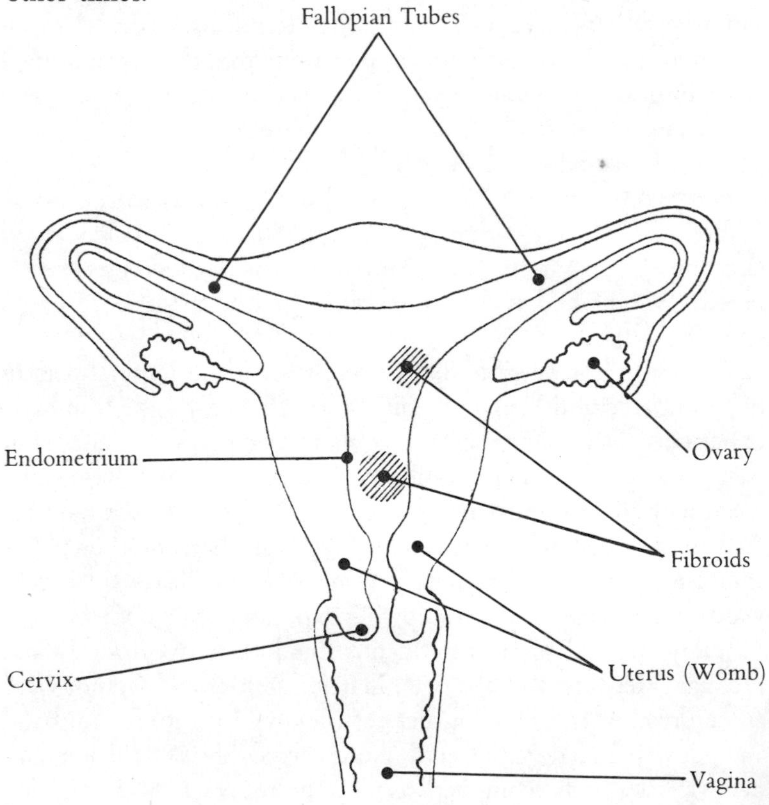

Diagram 1: Common Fibroid Sites

The link between oestrogen and fibroid growth means that very often, after the natural menopause when oestrogen levels fall, the fibroids shrink.

Fibroids vary from the size of a small pellet to a grapefruit or as big as a football. They are often mistakenly confused with cancer but they have nothing to do with cancer, nor do they spread outside the uterus. This means that they do not always need to be removed.

Sometimes a patient may be advised to have large fibroids removed, even though she is not experiencing any ill effects, in the concern that if they do grow larger, serious complications will occur later on.

Problems tend to occur when fibroids grow large and press on the surrounding pelvic structures, causing trouble with the bladder, bowel or rectum. They may also grow large enough to interfere with sexual intercourse, making it a painful and uncomfortable experience.

Very rarely the fibroid itself can become painful. It grows out into the uterus like a mushroom and then twists round on its own stem, causing acute pain and cutting off its own blood supply. As a result it will die and, if not removed by surgery, the accumulation of calcium salts over the years will result in a hard mass called a calcified fibroid or 'womb stone'.

Fibroids can make life troublesome in other ways when they are sited under the womb lining (endometrium), expanding it and causing heavy bleeding during menstruation. Although they do not interrupt the regularity of periods, their existence often means increased blood loss and perhaps anaemia.

Another cause for concern is a *fibrous polyp*. This occurs on a fibroid as it grows with its stem into the cavity of the womb. The womb responds by trying to eject the alien object. This rejection process makes itself felt by painful cramps especially during periods. Sometimes the uterus (womb) manages to push the fibroid further down towards the opening of the cervix. The stem gets longer and may even stretch open the cervix. As a result you may be in continuous pain and suffer irregular bleeding from the surface tissue of what is now a fibroid polyp.

Myomectomy

A myomectomy operation is the removal of fibroid swellings *and nothing else*. It is a difficult operation because it involves shelling out the growths and patching up the spaces that have been left.

This kind of repair is carried out when a woman still wishes to become pregnant and therefore wants to leave her womb intact, but at the same time wants the cause of her complaint removed.

The trouble is, myomectomy cannot effectively control excessive bleeding. And even if a patient is submitted for a myomectomy, it may after all become necessary to remove the womb totally, in order to control blood loss.

It is further discouraged as an operation because pregnancy after a myomectomy is fraught with all kinds of hazards. Furthermore, the relief of such symptoms as painful or heavy periods is not necessarily improved after myomectomy and the fibroids may even grow again.

Endometriosis

Researching this book, we discovered why endometriosis is called by some 'an enigmatic disorder'. Some literature states that endometriosis is common, some that it is a rare condition, and some literature didn't mention it at all! This obvious confusion could be because nobody in the medical profession knows exactly *why* it occurs.

There does, however, seem to be agreement on what happens: the cells which form the endometrium (womb lining) develop outside their normal location. This means that, instead of being part of the tissue of the lining, the cells form little clusters outside the uterus; they may invade the wall of the uterus or be found scattered throughout the pelvic cavity.

Sometimes they are found on the ligaments supporting the uterus, or between the uterus and the bowel. Apparently, more rarely, this tissue can be found in other parts of the body as well, including the lungs or inside the bowel. The growth of this tissue in the wrong place is called *endometriosis*. The development of the tissue in itself need cause no symptoms. On the other hand, it can be the cause of extremely severe and disabling pain. The reason for this is that these cells are made up of endometrial tissue so they must behave in the way they have been programmed.

You will remember that, as the level of hormones rises and falls each month, the tissue thickens and then breaks down in response. Even though these renegade cells are not in the correct place they still follow the same programme, so each month in response to the hormones, they grow during the menstrual cycle and die off during menstruation. When this happens within the womb, the blood can escape. But when these cells are growing elsewhere in the pelvis, the blood has nowhere to go. This causes swelling and pain, and as the accumulated blood degenerates, the growths inflame the surrounding area and scar tissue can form.

Sometimes the growths rupture, which spreads more cells to new areas to repeat the same process. Small blood-filled cysts can form on the ovaries or in any of the pelvic tissue around the bladder, bowel or uterus. Various organs can get stuck together (adhesions) and this will interfere with the normal functioning of the bladder, bowel or intestines if the growths are in these areas.

Although this is the basic pattern of endometriosis, the experience of it is wide-ranging. This will depend on the physical extent of the disease. It may affect one small part of a woman's body, or spread throughout her pelvis. Sometimes it may last for a short while and disappear without treatment. At other times a woman with endometriosis may suffer most of her reproductive life.

At the very worst, you can be in severe pain during menstruation; find sexual intercourse extremely painful; be subject to heavy or irregular bleeding; notice disruption of normal bowel functions; be prone to constant tiredness; and as a result some women find themselves infertile.

Endometriosis is hard to diagnose, especially in the early stages. Often the only certain way to detect the disease is a minor operation called a *laparoscopy*, where the surgeon makes a tiny incision through the abdomen, and pumps it up with carbon dioxide gas so that the organs are more easily seen through the laparoscope (a telescopic tube with a light in it).

Adenomyosis

This is another form of endometriosis. The renegade tissue develops in the usual way, but this time it buries itself into the wall of the uterus (womb), causing the walls of the uterus to expand every time a woman has a period; again the blood cannot escape, but continues to accumulate inside. Very painful periods, heavy bleeding and severe back pain are experienced by those suffering from adenomyosis.

Among the women interviewed, Margaret alone reported that she had a hysterectomy because of endometriosis; Nikki had adenomyosis. But it could well have contributed to the symptoms described by other women without their being aware of it, especially as so few were told after their operations what had in fact been found to be wrong.

Pelvic inflammatory disease (PID)

Common infections in the pelvis affect many women but most of these are not serious. They can be irritating and uncomfortable but are contained at the entrance of or inside the vagina.

Of course, it is important to treat the infections but grave problems only occur when the infection affects the uterus, the Fallopian tubes or the ovaries.

These kinds of infections are less common but more serious in their consequences. The tragedy is that symptoms often go unacknowledged and therefore the disease continues undiagnosed in many women, with the result that effective treatment is not given in time to stop the disease spreading and causing irreversible damage.

Infections can occur after childbirth or abortion; they may be the result of sexually transmitted diseases such as gonorrhoea; use of an IUD coil; they can spread from infections in other organs such as appendix, urinary tract or the infection can be carried in the blood. The Fallopian tubes are particularly vulnerable to infection. Salpingitis (infection of the Fallopian tubes) is a common disease of the pelvis and if it persists, abcesses can form on the Fallopian tubes with the result that both tubes and ovaries can become scarred, and possibly lead to infertility.

Symptoms of pelvic inflammatory disease are severe – abdominal pain, a high temperature and an offensive-smelling discharge from the vagina. You may experience pain during intercourse or menstruation, your cycle may become less regular and your blood loss heavier.

When infections become chronic, as in Jenny's case mentioned earlier, there is a risk of serious illness. A doctor may well recommend the removal of the damaged organs as the only way of containing the disease. Surgery is often sought because the recurring infection causes so much pain and disorder. But surgery only applies in the most severe cases. If antibiotics are given early on and consistently until all signs of the infection have cleared, then a cure by drugs is possible.

This may involve a course of antibiotics which could run into months or even a couple of years, and this is where a choice has to be made between long-term drug therapy, with the prospect of avoiding hysterectomy altogether, and destroying the infection more directly by surgical removal of the diseased parts – ovaries, Fallopian tubes, uterus.

Cancer

For women who have a malignant disease (cancerous tumour) of the cervix, the uterus, the ovary or the endometrium (womb lining), hysterectomy is performed to save the woman's life. The diseased parts are removed before the disease can spread.

Surgery will depend on how advanced the cancer is discovered to be. If it is detected early (at the pre-invasive stage), cancer cells have formed within the uterus lining but not spread anywhere else. If it is left undetected, the cancer may have spread into the uterus or outside and into the pelvic area.

Depending on where the cancer cells are, the lining of the uterus alone will be removed, or the uterus in total, especially if the patient is experiencing severe menstrual pain or bleeding.

If the cancer is discovered later on and has already spread to the uterus, then surgery is definitely necessary and the uterus will be removed. But the extent of surgery required will vary with the kind of cancer found and how far it has spread.

Of course, patients may wish to have treatment other than surgery for cancer, which may include radiation which attacks cancer cells, or drugs containing substances that prevent growth of more cells and sometimes hormone treatment can be used to check the spread of cancer.

Some women are discovered to have cancer in one or both ovaries, in which case a hysterectomy including the removal of both ovaries is advisable in order to contain the disease.

Prolapsed womb

One last common reason for hysterectomy is a prolapse. This describes not a disease, but a structural fault in our anatomy. The word prolapse means the displacement of any organ from its normal position.

Chart 1: Gynaecological Cancer Sites

Type	Treatment
Most common: Cancer of the cervix	Burning/freezing (cauterizing) the cervix; biopsy (small amount of cervical tissue removed); radiotherapy to destroy the malignant cells; perhaps hysterectomy if larger area of cervix is affected. Uterus and cervix removed.
Second most common: Cancer of the endometrium	D & C; then hysterectomy (uterus, Fallopian tubes and top inch of vagina removed), plus radiotherapy before or after operation, plus oestrogen/progestogen combination hormone therapy may prevent cancer returning.
Third most common: Cancer of the ovaries	Hysterectomy (removal of uterus, Fallopian tubes, ovaries) or chemotherapy (use of chemical substances which kill the disease without injuring the patient).
Very rare: Cancer of the Fallopian tube	Hysterectomy (removal of Fallopian tubes, probably ovaries, uterus and cervix.
Still rarer: Cancer of the uterine muscle	Hysterectomy (as directly above).
Even rarer still: Cancerous fibroid	Hysterectomy (as directly above).

Chart 2:
Reasons for Hysterectomy – Type – How Soon You Will Recover

Symptoms	**Type of operation required**	**Recovery rate**
Anything other than Cancer	*Subtotal:* removal of uterus only; cervix left in place. *OR* *Total:* removal of uterus and cervix.	Most rapid: 6-12 weeks. Most rapid: 6-12 weeks.
Cysts; pre-invasive (early) cancer; severe pelvic inflammatory disease; ovaries no longer functioning i.e. post menopause	*Bi-lateral Salpingo oopherectomy:* removal of uterus, Fallopian tubes, ovaries.	Rapid: 10-12 weeks
Spreading cancer	*Extended or Wertheim:* removal of uterus, cervix, part of vagina; Fallopian tubes and all the lymph nodes and vessels plus part of the cardinal and utero sacral ligaments. More dissection necessary therefore more haemorrhage is likely.	Least rapid: 4 months or longer.
Prolapse: uterus has dropped	Vaginal hysterectomy removal of uterus via the vagina.	Most rapid: 6-12 weeks.

REMEMBER: CANCER CAN BE CURED – The earlier it is detected through regular cervical smear tests, the greater the chance of a 100 per cent cure.

A prolapse of the womb means that the womb has dropped due to a weakening of the ligaments that support it. This puts pressure on the bladder in front and the rectum behind. As the vaginal walls weaken under the pressure of the dropped womb, the bladder and rectum push in on the vagina from front and back.

If the uterus (womb) is healthy, removal is not necessary and 'vaginal repair' is carried out. This is really plastic surgery of the vagina. The extra slack skin is taken up and the supporting tissue of the vaginal walls are lifted and strengthened. In this way women can continue to have periods and pregnancy is still possible.

However, if a woman has had menstrual problems then the uterus (womb) can be removed and the vagina repaired at the same time. This usually means that a vaginal hysterectomy will be performed (see Chapter 5). This operation is similarly carried out in cases of older women whose wombs have dropped because the supports have thinned due to lower levels of female sex hormones – oestrogen and progesterone. Again the womb would have to be removed through the vagina.

You will see from the charts on pages 34 and 35 that all these different symptoms require different kinds of surgery.

4

Talking it Through

All the women interviewed were married at the time of their hysterectomy, apart from Margaret who was separated from her husband, and Louise who was living with her partner and later married.

Many researchers agree that the attitude of the partner is important to rapid recovery. Even so, few husbands show any interest in what is going to happen to their wives when a hysterectomy is recommended.

'Hysterectomy brings about a fundamental change in a woman, like having a baby: she needs support from her partner. Although partners may be involved in childbirth these days, they are *not* involved in hysterectomy.' (*Gynae*)

One of the causes of this general lack of concern is the fact that hysterectomy is part of the reproductive process and like many other aspects of a woman's sexuality – menstruation, contraception, childbirth, menopause – it is felt to be 'women's business' and therefore out of bounds to men.

In our own and other cultures, menstrual blood is a taboo which elicits anxiety. By association, excessive bleeding which prompts many women to seek hysterectomy is just another gynaecological symptom which men don't really want to know about.

A husband's involvement in hysterectomy will depend on how sympathetic or involved he is in the symptoms which bring his wife to the gynaecologist. 'If she wakes up in bed and there is a pool of blood, and he's covered in blood too, they have to go to the bathroom and wash themselves down. If they can do that and laugh about it, that's fine. But usually she's ashamed and he is appalled.' (*Gynae*)

Apart from particular hang-ups, his involvement will obviously also depend on what their relationship has been like up until then:

how they express their love and interest in each other and how he feels about his own and her sexuality. Another problem is lack of information.

'Husbands are often more ignorant than their wives. They might come up to the desk and say the word *hysterectomy* but they don't know what that is really. I always say "Yes, she has had her womb removed."' (*Staff Nurse*)

A man may be worried about how his wife will change; whether she will become depressed or 'emotional'. An apparently common concern is how much the operation will affect their sex-life.

Resuming sexual relations after surgery is important, but we have decided to explore this in a separate chapter (see Chapter 10, Sex and Sexuality) because although sex can be an integral part of a relationship, we feel there are other important issues to be considered: for example, involvement in the actual decision to have a hysterectomy and the provision of care and support while his wife is in hospital both immediately she comes home and longer term care.

Sharing the decision

Are partners involved in discussions with the consultant beforehand? Is the decision shared or is it felt to be the woman's sole responsibility?

'The fact that it was a hysterectomy was not discussed fully, nor the implications. J was not involved in the discussion [with the doctor] or the decision. (*Jenny*)

'My husband was involved to a certain extent, although I made the final decision. I discussed it with him and he said "I'll go along with whatever you want, it's your body."' (*Sally*)

'My husband said, "Well if that's what they say you've got to have, you'd better have it."' (*Carole*)

'He wasn't involved at all. It was my decision and he knew about it from his medical training, but I don't think it concerned him much.' (*Elaine*)

'He said, "Obviously, you've got to go and have something done," but he didn't want to be involved all that much.' (*Fiona*)

The implications of hysterectomy as an end to the possibility of pregnancy were crucial to the attitudes of three of the partners. Ellen's husband encouraged her: 'My husband didn't want any more children, even though I did, and he didn't like my being so tired all the time. He felt if I had it, it would be an improvement.'

Jenny's partner, too, welcomed hysterectomy in a long-standing conflict: 'He didn't want children, so a hysterectomy was a relief to him. It meant that it need no longer be an issue between us.'

For Louise it was the reverse: 'He desperately wanted a child. It had to be a boy to carry the name over. I felt very inadequate after the operation because I couldn't give him the one thing he wanted.'

The prospect of hysterectomy was described as a welcome relief to two other men, but this was specifically relief from their wives' long-standing symptoms and suffering. A woman's physical symptoms can have a disruptive effect on all those around her. 'He was relieved that what I was like, and becoming, was going to stop. He was relieved that I was going to be in control of my own body. Because, honestly, he couldn't have gone on living with me. He said, "I just can't go on with you like this, it's impossible." For M to say that, it takes quite a lot.' (*Jean*)

And although Sally's husband had recognized that it was primarily her decision, that she was the one who was suffering, he added that he was suffering too, but in a different way. 'Which he was. It was affecting the whole family. My two children were not old enough to understand what was going on but things were very strained at home.'

In contrast to the general assumption that men don't want to be involved, both Jean and Sally found great support from their husbands, in doing so. Jean had been given a PMT chart, which helped her identify a pattern to her moods, backache and tiredness and so on. This helped them both to see what was going to happen and when. This enabled them to cope better and certainly involved him in the eventual decision to have the operation.

Some wives keep it all a secret; their husbands don't even know when they have a period. 'I had to warn him: I'd say "it's the time, I feel strung up and I feel bad." If it was ovulation pain, he had to know because if he saw me lying down and unable to move, he would have been upset and frightened and not know what to do. So I had to involve him.' (*Sally*)

Angela's husband was the key person in her decision to finally go ahead after hanging on for two years. 'What really made me change my mind was when I went to Ireland for a wedding. I got off the plane and my husband hadn't seen me objectively for a long time. He came to meet me and said "What on earth is the matter with you? You look terrible." And it was just the usual, so I thought, "Gosh, if I look that bad perhaps I'd better have the operation." He was anxious that I looked so ill and if this was the answer, I should get on with it. So I went back to the doctor and was in within a fortnight.'

Only two women reported that their husbands had actually seen the consultant themselves. Celia's husband was a dentist with some medical knowledge but, after discussing it with her, still took the time to see the consultant afterwards.

Sandra's husband was in hospital for a heart operation at the same time as she was having her hysterectomy. He decided to see the doctor himself, to find out what they could or could not do: 'We wanted to go on holiday and to know if we could travel. He said, "I want to know what's happened. I don't want to get it second-hand from you."'

After the operation a woman needs a supportive person around in hospital and during recovery. None of the women interviewed reported any lack of concern from partners while they were in hospital, apart from Elaine whose doctor/husband was 'busy elsewhere'.

The importance of talking beforehand is not only to know what will happen but to be able to make adequate plans for the recovery period. Some partners may understand the full implications. 'He was very supportive about my having surgery and not being fit afterwards for a time,' said Jenny. But others may not know just how much help their wives need. 'I did sometimes think he was a little bit uncaring afterwards, when it was painful. He expected rather too much of me. He wasn't sexually demanding, but physically, doing things around the house when I was still sore.' (*Fiona*)

Sometimes this lack of care stems from not having discussed things properly beforehand, and not making plans together for the recovery period, especially if there are young children around. 'Everything should be well organized at home before the patient is admitted. I don't think the husband should have too much pressure looking after the children. Sometimes the younger men can get very temperamental. After a week of looking after the kids they've had it! They often come in and take it out on the wife. Nine times out of ten the wife is in tears because she feels guilty. I think his duty is to come to see his wife every day. To sit and talk with her and not tell her all the problems of what's going on at home. Another member of the family or even a good neighbour can take some of these pressures off him, so that they can go through this time together. I think that is very important.' (*Staff Nurse*)

'Ideally, he should come and help with the decision; with the plans for recovery; he should come to the operating theatre and wait outside. But they never do that.' (*Gynae*)

We started off this chapter by saying that the very nature of this operation makes it difficult for many men to feel it is their concern, or to feel free to ask questions. Many are reluctant to make an enquiry and hesitate to get involved. Although some men are no doubt happier like this, it seems that even those who would like to be more involved are discouraged from doing so by their partners and also by the majority of the medical profession.

'I didn't talk about it to him because he wasn't interested to know the details.' (*Fiona*)

'Because it was a charged issue, I may not have given him any information. But he didn't seek any information from the consultant himself.' (*Jenny*)

'We don't instruct the sister on the ward to talk to the partner because we generally assume that the men don't want to be involved.' (*Gynae*)

It seems we are in danger of a chicken and egg situation arising, whereby although many medical practitioners agree that husbands should be more informed, they don't provide the facility, which means that the men are left uninformed and are then assumed to be uninterested.

It appears that the onus is on the individual man to make an approach: 'The partner will have to make it very clear that he wants to be more closely involved or wants more information.' The gynaecologist went on to say that if he did want to find out more about what was going on, an appointment could be made with the houseman. The problem is 'the houseman is the least experienced of the team, and might not give a balanced view or allay the husband's fears, because he might have the same hang-ups and fears as the husband.' (*Gynae*) So where do we go from here? The gynaecologist recommends that 'in an ideal world the spouse should go and see the consultant, sit down for twenty minutes, with or without the patient, who will explain what is going on. But I don't see that happening in the present organization of health care.'

In view of this, as Sally and Jean demonstrated, the best way to overcome this barrier is to make sure you talk to your partner yourself, and if possible ask your partner to go to the consultant with you.

Sharing the whole experience in this way from the beginning can deepen the trust between you. Another reason for keeping it all to ourselves is because we don't want to alarm or upset the other person. But however difficult, it is precisely these things which are important to share.

Two years after the event Jean still regretted not having told her husband about the possibility of her having cancer. She didn't take M to the clinic because she anticipated being told that she might have cancer.

'I didn't want to cause him unnecessary worry, and tell him about something that might not be there. The first he knew about it was when he signed the consent form. He said, "Why didn't you tell me you suspected cancer?" I think he eventually understood that I had to get myself together because I'm that sort of person, but he was terribly hurt that I didn't confide in him. I didn't want him to worry about *me* worrying about *it*. The trouble was that up until then we'd shared everything and helped each other out. He would never mention it but I don't think he's ever forgotten. I think it was a very silly thing to do.' Nevertheless, their relationship proved strong enough to cope with the crisis.

This was true for most of the women we interviewed. Although we did hear reports of husbands leaving their wives due to emotional complications following hysterectomy, this didn't happen to any of the women in our group, with the exception of Louise. 'Eventually we split up three years after, because it would keep coming up that I couldn't give him the child he wanted.'

Being able to anticipate hurdles is better than being taken by surprise. It's better to know what *could* happen even if things turn out better than expected. In anticipation of how Angela might feel on her return, her husband planned a welcome-home surprise: 'People had told him that you are often very emotionally upset afterwards; so while I was in hospital he went out and bought a new bedroom suite, so that I would have a new bedroom to come back to. As it turned out, I wasn't a bit emotional, but the bedroom suite was still a wonderful surprise.'

We must not make the mistake of assuming that every woman who has a hysterectomy has a husband. Many women experience this operation as single, in a relationship with a woman, divorced, or widowed. In these situations close friends or relatives can be an enormous source of care and understanding, both practically and emotionally; especially if the person is a woman who has undergone the same operation. And in focusing on husbands as partners in this chapter, we do not want to underestimate the vital role that friends play whether you are married or single, before, during and after the whole experience.

5
Making a Decision

'Don't have it done until you are absolutely sure that it is the right decision. Don't be badgered into it by anyone else. Don't have it done unless you are 100 per cent sure you want it done.' (*Celia*)

Unless you have cancer, you always have a choice whether or not to have a hysterectomy, and even with cancer, there is a range of alternative treatments to surgery. If you are investigating the possibility of hysterectomy, it's likely you consider it a solution to unwanted symptoms.

The two main areas of concern are whether hysterectomy is in fact the answer, and whether losing your womb will have any significance to you.

Is hysterectomy the answer?

Discounting cancer, if there is something physically wrong with your womb, there are alternative treatments.

Fibroids can be removed by myomectomy; a prolapsed womb can be repaired; endometriosis, heavy bleeding and PMS can be relieved with hormonal medication or even herbal remedies. The efficacy of alternative treatments to major surgery will obviously depend on the severity of the symptoms.

Age is another important factor. For example, if you are close to your menopause and have fibroids, the symptoms will automatically be alleviated with the natural change in your hormonal levels. Fibroids are believed to be dependent on oestrogen for their growth. It follows that when the oestrogen level falls after the menopause, the fibroids will shrink and the symptoms will disappear of their own accord. To prevent anaemia, supplementary medication may be necessary, but you may not need to undergo surgery.

Unnecessary surgery can be avoided by understanding that hysterectomy is sometimes a physical solution to an emotional problem; that heavy bleeding and other symptoms associated with premenstrual tension may be caused not by any fault in the functioning of the womb, but by external stress in your life.

Under all sorts of stress 'the endometrium responds like the skin on your face by blushing.' (*Gynae*) This blushing continues if the reason for your anxiety persists – bereavement, job loss, difficulties in a personal relationship, avoiding sexual contact, emotional conflict, unexpressed anger – bodily changes which upset the hormonal balance can all precipitate and disturb the menstrual pattern and affect the blood loss.

Unfortunately, most medical professionals are insufficiently alert to the correlation between emotional stress and physical symptoms. Therefore it is important for a woman to ask herself honestly if there is any possibility that her symptoms could be more directly dealt with by confronting the stressful situation. She may just require sympathetic professional help to do this, rather than undergo surgery.

The significance of your womb

The first question to ask yourself is an obvious one. How do you feel about not having any more children? This can be relatively easily answered. All the women we interviewed except for Louise, were very clear about this one particular point.

Sometimes a woman views her womb as a mechanical part of her body, a significant mechanical part, but one which can be taken away without problems. 'They're only removing the bag in which the embryo grows. They're not taking anything else away.' (*Fiona*)

'As far as I'm concerned it had done a good job. Like an old coat really, I'd worn it and enjoyed it and I'd got my children, so it was of no use to me any more.' (*Celia*)

'It was more than useless, it was a damned nuisance!' (*Elaine*)

However, for other women the womb has a less obvious significance. In some cultures fertility and womanhood are very closely connected and, for this reason, women resist losing their wombs and hysterectomy. In our own culture too, this attitude is evident.

Hysterectomy is regarded as a 'failure, as an interference with the expression of the femininity and their womanhood. They *hate* it. I think some women regard it as one step closer to the grave and their eternal reckoning. This attitude prevails among old and young women. I recently spoke to an elderly lady with a prolapsed womb. We sat down and talked. She really doesn't want a hysterectomy. Even though she's seventy-two, she really feels it is a destruction of her femininity.' (*Gynae*)

Ellen came to terms with it afterwards, but feared something similar: 'My womb did have some symbolic feeling for me. I thought I might lose the ability to have children *and* my femininity at the same time. I know now I only lost the one.'

In the course of our interviews we talked to Suzanne, who had been advised to have a hysterectomy by her consultant because of fibroids, and consequent heavy bleeding. 'It's an inconvenience, a real nuisance and always happens at the wrong time. But I've chosen to put up with the inconvenience rather than go through the trauma of an operation for various reasons.' She feared it would affect her sexuality and how she felt about her body.

'I've had four children, so my uterus is emotionally very important to me. I can't explain it. It's just terribly important to me that I have my uterus. It's so daft really because I don't need it. I was happily sterilized five years ago. I'm fifty, so there's no way I'm going to have another child. But it's that knowledge that hysterectomy will somehow take away my feeling fertile. It's not rational, in fact it's illogical. My head says "Your womb's redundant, it's served you very well. You have four beautiful children and you don't need it," but my body says "Yes you do!"' (*Suzanne*)

Taking all this into account, you may still decide that hysterectomy is the best solution for you. Before reaching the final decision here are some questions you might like the consultant to answer:

- Are the ovaries going to be removed at all or damaged in any way so that premature menopause can be expected?
- Is the vagina going to be shortened?
- What special provision is going to be made for relief of pain following the operation?
- What are the specific complications?
- What provisions are made for these complications to be minimal or avoided altogether?

- How soon will recovery be?
- What long term disabilities might there be?
- What help can be arranged during the convalescent period?

If you don't have cancer and you are in a position to choose *not* to have a hysterectomy, you will be interested to know that our gynaecologist stated quite clearly:

'I have never seen anybody die from refusing to have a hysterectomy.' (*Gynae*)

Preparing Yourself

If you do decide to go ahead with hysterectomy, physical and mental preparation is highly recommended.

'You must be as fit as you can before the operation. If you have a choice in the date, have it when you are feeling good. It is important to prepare yourself physically with your diet, and not be overweight. Although good health is important at all times, it is particularly so when you are going to have some physical trauma. You need to be fit and in tip-top condition. You must also completely come to terms with it mentally.' (*Elaine*)

'Get yourself physically and mentally as fit as you can before embarking on the operation. If you've lost your job or your husband has left you, or you're low anyway, *don't* go ahead with it. If it is not an emergency and you have the chance to decide, it is important to take the time to think about it.' (*Sally*)

Our gynaecologist recommended preparing yourself by understanding what was going to happen, and allowing for a longer convalescence than the GP or consultant has advised. He also said it is not a good idea to be very overweight, because surplus fat makes the surgery technically more difficult.

Domestic arrangements are also very important. 'Plan well in advance, make sure everything is in order as far as the family goes, so you don't have to worry.' (*Sally*)

'Practically I prepared myself well. I organized surgery for a convenient time in between jobs, and I arranged my domestic duties so that I wouldn't have a great deal to do.' (*Jenny*)

Several women felt it was a good idea to talk about it to as many people as possible. In this way you could accustom yourself to the idea. Talking to women who have been through hysterectomy themselves can be reassuring. (See Further Information, page 134, for details of the Hysterectomy Support Group.)

From the professional viewpoint, the Staff Nurse recommended 'more leaflets, drawings of women's bodies, something simple nothing technical, should be available in hospital out-patients, gynaecology units, GP surgeries.' She also recommended more contact with the GP and the hospital before patients are admitted: 'I'd love them to come and spend a couple of hours on the ward beforehand; case the environment and meet the nurses who will look after them.' But alas, that remains a fantasy as is the consultant's idea of a patient's 'friend'.

'When the patient clocks in to the hospital clerk, we need someone to be allocated to them who will stay with them all the time they are in hospital. When any discussion takes place between the patient and doctor, the "friend" can ask questions on the patient's behalf. I think this would diffuse the tremendous emotional anxieties and disorientation people feel in hospital.' (*Gynae*) And although this is wishful thinking at the moment, he added, 'I'm going to employ a counsellor at my hospital, whose job it will be to talk to patients as they come in.'

Some women need the time to adjust to the idea before and *after* the operation. Even though this part of your body has become identified with pain and inconvenience, it can be important to acknowledge or 'mourn' the loss of an integral part of our bodies and our lives. This may mean no more than allowing a time for transition between the past and the future; between the old you and the new you, and recognizing that perhaps the uterus is more than just a bit of disposable tissue.

As we described earlier, the uterus can be profoundly associated with our feelings of being a woman. For some women, hysterectomy is the very last resort and they can be reluctant to accept it as a final solution, even though all other treatment has failed to alleviate the distressing symptoms. For these women our gynaecologist described hysterectomy as 'a treatment of despair'. In situations like this, a time for mourning is essential.

Finally, we recommend that you find some way of giving yourself a personal treat.

'So much of me didn't want to have the operation so I pampered that bit of me. I thought, "If I have to have it, I want everything to go easily." I elected to go privately. I bought myself an expensive pair of silk slippers, so every time I got out of bed and slid into them, I felt like a million dollars.' (*Ellen*)

6
The Professionals

A woman's perception of her hysterectomy will be shaped by her contact with professionals involved along the way; from her very first consultation with the GP, through to her referral to a consultant gynaecologist; throughout her pre- and post-operative care in hospital at the hands of the nursing staff, to her eventual return home and subsequent check-ups, and her ultimate complete recovery.

A large part of the responsibility for whether a woman's experience is positive or negative, depends on the particular professionals she has the good luck or misfortune to encounter. It depends whether their approach is sympathetic or dismissive; whether adequate information is given or withheld; whether or not they are technically proficient and the hospital facilities up to scratch or below par.

Writing this book, we have come to the distressing conclusion that whether or not you have a happy hysterectomy is a question of sheer luck, and that there can never be a guarantee of carefree passage. In order to avoid potential pitfalls, we thought it best to start by considering the different roles of the GP, specialist and the nurse, so that with a more thorough understanding of how their roles are defined, any prospective patient can make the best use of their expertise and power, and the facilities available to her.

The General Practitioner

The GP is the first professional with whom you are likely to discuss your symptoms, and the GP's attitude at this time is significant. 'I would really have liked to sit down and have a good conversation about what would happen before and after. My GP tried to pacify me by saying that thousands of women have it done every year. "You're worrying yourself about nothing." That was it.' (*Carole*)

Jean was also unhappy about her GP's attitude to her description of her symptoms, although he agreed to refer her for a second opinion. 'I read my doctor's letter and even though he has known me for years, he was very sceptical and had written, "This patient has asked to be referred to you. I think she is worried about having a D and C." I felt furious. Nobody was taking *me*, as a person, seriously.'

A particular GP's attitude can prove an obstacle or a help. Fiona tried unsuccessfully to persuade her GP that she wanted a hysterectomy for five years. 'Finally, I found a GP who was sympathetic, who said, "It's ridiculous that somebody should have to carry on like that just because of age."' (*Fiona*)

Our gynaecologist felt strongly about the GP's role as s/he is likely to be more familiar with the patient's circumstances; he believed the initial discussion was very significant.

'In an ideal world, the GP will realize that a hysterectomy is necessary and have said in the discussion with the patient, "I'm sending you to a gynaecologist who might suggest hysterectomy. What are your feelings about this?" The treatment options could then be fully explained.' (*Gynae*)

However, as Sandra said: 'It's just your hard luck if your GP is not interested in your particular illness.'

Even in a large team practice, you may be assigned to a GP with little knowledge or enthusiasm for gynaecological problems. Therefore 'women's complaints' may not be considered very important.

According to the gynaecologist, the reality is 'that the GP is not sure of the diagnosis and too busy doing other things.' He described a typical interaction between GP and patient: '"You've got problems with your periods? Well, what's your name, age and your address? Right, I'll send you off to the hospital because they are better at it and I can't do a vaginal examination here. I've got a room full of patients outside waiting. You give this letter to the receptionist, she'll put your NHS number on it. Oh, you know it, good! Send it off to the hospital and you'll see one of the gynaecologists. Which one? Well, I don't know. One of them has a long waiting list, the other two don't, and you want this done quickly." The letter arrives saying: "Dear Gynae, please see Mrs X.

Period problems. Leave it up to you."' (*Gynae*)

This brings us to the key function of the GP's role. It is possible to survive a dismissive attitude but it is *crucial* to be referred to a surgeon who is competent. Patients on the NHS are very much restricted to the luck of the draw as to who happens to be a gynaecologist in their hospital catchment area. Therefore the GP's choice is vital to the successful outcome of the operation as patients do not have access to relevant information. At this point you are entirely in your GP's hands, and yet as the gynaecologist says: 'The GP may not even know to whom s/he is sending you. In wanting the problem solved, s/he sends you to the nearest or quickest who can see you and may not mind if you are seen by an assistant rather than the consultant in person. Sometimes who you end up with is dependent on the hospital administration. The GP writes to the department of the hospital and a clerk slots you into someone's list. Usually, NHS patients accept that decision and stay with that surgeon or a member of that team.' (*Gynae*)

We asked how you spot a good surgeon when you see one. 'The surgeon's training and qualifications can be discovered in the Medical Directory/Register [available in any local reference library], but your GP should choose the surgeon carefully by referring you to a consultant whose wounds heal. It's like gardening. Good surgeons have perfected a technique which involves a minimum amount of tissue handling, which results in rapid recovery. There are some surgeons whose wounds heal, and there are some who are very clever but who always get into complications – the wounds get infected, there is a discharge, they break down. It all lies in the way you handle the tissue.' (*Gynae*)

How does the GP obtain the necessary information?

'Sometimes by reputation: s/he can phone the registrar at the hospital and ask for an opinion, or can phone the surgeon's colleagues and check on her/his reputation. The GP can also learn from patients previously referred to a particular surgeon. The GP is the the one to get feedback. For example, "the surgeon wasn't very nice". Or "I've had a discharge for a month." Or "there was a problem in the hospital because they had to re-stitch me." Or "I never saw the consultant after the operation." Or "none of the Juniors spoke English."' (*Gynae*)

In this way a GP can build a profile of a particular surgeon's skills and attitudes, in order to do the best for the patient. Whether it is a vaginal or abdominal hysterectomy, the GP can recommend the best surgeon available. And if there is any doubt as to the necessity for hysterectomy, send the patient to a consultant gynaecologist who is not just going to whip it all out on principle.

'The GP must choose according to whether a surgeon is kind and sympathetic; whose wounds heal; who will give a fair opinion; who will be able to get the patient into a nice hospital, within a reasonable time. If the GP has done her/his homework, fine.' (*Gynae*)

The GP's role is not only confined to referrals before the operation. Apparently, some private patients have the advantage of having their GPs present in the operating theatre: 'S/he takes the role of first assistant. It's very nice when they come, because they can hold the patient's hand in the anaesthetic department. The patient knows s/he's there. It's super. It doesn't happen very often because they are too busy.' (*Gynae*)

For most of us, the GP resumes responsibility on our return home from hospital. Rehabilitation of patients is something consultants at the hospital know little about. 'It's something we don't touch on at all really. We tend to leave it to the GP. I would expect the patient to be seeing her GP weekly following her discharge from hospital.' (*Gynae*)

Sandra's 'superb' GP appeared the day she came out of hospital, but as a Health Visitor, she recognized that this was rare. 'Most patients will not receive a post-op visit because most GPs won't know their patients have had the operation. They write the letter to make the initial appointment three months ahead, but unless you go and see your GP regularly, letters don't get written and you could have been home ten days before the letter gets back to the GP.'

It's a pity if a GP assumes that, once the referral is made, her/his responsibility to the patient ends. 'I would have liked someone to talk to after, so I could tell them how I was feeling. There was no one I could talk to, not even my GP. As far as he was concerned, it was finished. He had done his part. The rest of it was up to me to get over it. In my own time and in my own way. I found it very, very hard to accept his attitude as well.' (*Louise*)

We fully realize that many GPs are struggling to provide an adequate service to their patients within the constraints of the NHS, and that there is little 'extra' time available. However, it does seem imperative that the GP chooses wisely to whom patients are referred for operations, rather than leaving it to chance. Repercussions from any operation can last a lifetime.

In addition, patients themselves have a responsibility 'to always go back to the GP and say what they felt about it all. "It was smashing; fantastic; I'm fine. Thank you for choosing that surgeon." Or, "Wasn't there someone else you could have sent me to?" The patient's personal post-operative report is vital.' (*Gynae*)

The Consultant

'I regard all my patients as slightly sacred in that they are your mother and your sister rolled into one, and I behave as someone I would like to look after my wife and my daughter. That's an expression of my relationship with my patients.' (*Gynae*)

All but one of the women interviewed saw a male gynaecologist. This is typical and understandable as women are still very much in the minority in gynaecology, as in many other professions. Although we quote the experiences of being seen by male consultants, we believe attitudes and treatment are the same, whether the consultant is a man or a woman.

A popular belief about male gynaecologists is that they choose to specialize in gynaecology because they either adore women or they hate them; their treatment of their patients will vary accordingly.

Our gynaecologist suggested another pragmatic reason: 'There are gynaecologists who choose gynaecology not because they have any sympathy for women, but because obstetrics is the first subject in the under-graduate curriculum. They take it up because they are practical. They love doing something with their hands for the first time, and taking responsibility for patients. Then they find to their surprise, when they go into it further, there's a woman at the other end.' (*Gynae*)

He admitted that some gynaecologists could be cruel to their patients but felt that the hostility expressed to some women by some male consultants wasn't always due to a basic heartlessness. He believed it was due to 'An unidentified crisis concerning the patient's sexuality and their own sexuality, which expresses itself in antagonism, intolerance and a lack of sympathy.'

There is probably another reason which applies to both male and female medical professionals of all kinds: an inability to admit to mistakes, to ignorance and to human limitations. Faced with a patient for whom they can do nothing more, a deep sense of inadequacy and helplessness can often become distorted into an abrupt and dismissive manner. This can be easily perceived by the patient as hostile and uncaring.

Most women have experienced being on the receiving end of harsh treatment by medical professionals at some time or other. But we also know that it varies with the individual consultant.

The consultant's responsibility is the patient's care – how much that care will be manifest, depends largely on the individual's attitude to her/his work, the experience s/he has acquired and whether treatment is NHS or private.

'NHS clinic means sitting in a waiting room without tights, shoes or knickers. Lines and lines of women. I have never seen anything like that before. All with dressing gowns on, and skirts off, waiting, then wheeled into two consulting rooms, which the consultant travels between.' (*Jenny*)

'We are terribly busy. In the out-patients department I'll see fifteen to twenty new patients; ten follow-ups. My registrar will see 5 to 10 new patients, thirty follow-ups. My houseman will see thirty follow-ups. We start at 9.30 a.m. and we try to finish by 12.45. That's approximately two minutes for each patient. The NHS doesn't have sufficient time allotted for staff to sit down and talk to patients. I can't fulfil that role, even though I would like to, so I train my juniors to do that for me.' (*Gynae*)

'The contrast when I saw him in his private consulting rooms was amazing. His manner was equally charming NHS or private, but the difference in the amount of time he gave me [4 minutes–1 hour] was enormous.' (*Jenny*)

Whatever the context, meeting the consultant is a bit of a hurdle. Instead of the familiarity of the local surgery, you find yourself ushered in to see 'the expert' in a white coat. Interaction with any 'expert' can put us at an immediate disadvantage but flat on a table, legs apart, it is virtually impossible to retain a sense of dignity and self-confidence. It is easy to feel tongue-tied and intimidated. This is why the consultant's manner and attitude are so crucial and why sensitivity and respect are imperative.

It is important in discussing proposed surgery that the patient has some say in any decision concerning her body and that she is given the information she requires to help her make that decision. 'I had a surgeon who didn't have a sense of humour, but he was very good. He gave me lots of advice and information without any prompting. He told me what was going on and how things were going to happen.' (*Celia*)

'I felt the consultant was very good because he asked me "Do you *mind* having a hysterectomy?" and helped me look at my feelings about the prospect.' (*Margaret*)

Fiona's consultant was unusually forthcoming about sexual matters, and took time to explain fully what might happen. Several women reported being consulted about their feelings and being made to feel part of the decision.

Seeing the consultant in an NHS context varies with the gynaecological unit and the hospital. We've already described how Carole was given an ultimatum by her consultant while she was being examined in front of medical students. Her acceptance of his behaviour was because of the past associations. 'If I hadn't been with the consultant for so many years, and if he hadn't delivered my son, I would have been a bit more doubtful.' (*Carole*)

Louise's consultant gave her only half an hour to come to terms with what for her was an extremely difficult decision.

Jean caught the brunt of a consultant's impatience. 'When I first went to see the consultant, I saw him literally for 2 minutes. He said, "Right, we'll have you in for a D and C, and we'll let you know when." I said, "What about my backache?" His reply was, "Every woman your age [thirty-three] with three children has got to expect a bit of backache." I said, "I don't normally complain about anything, but it really is very painful. I can cope with it during the day by keeping busy, but I can't at night." He said, "Well that's it really, out!"' (*Jean*)

It is important to remember that because a woman feels very vulnerable at this time, her anxiety can make it difficult for her to listen and take things in clearly: 'When I saw the consultant at the beginning, he sat there after he'd examined me and said, "Have you got your holidays booked? I'm sure you'd like to get it over with, so we might as well do it now." I was convinced that this was a rather nonchalant way of telling me I was just about to die.' (*Margaret*)

Apart from the consultant's manner, the second vital factor is surgical *skill*. 'In gynaecology you can do something real and identifiable. You can deliver a baby modifying the delivery to minimize trauma for mother and baby. You can do an operation for which you need technical expertise and skill. You accept responsibility for doing that. If your wounds heal, and everything goes well, you can feel enormous satisfaction. If your wounds don't heal and things are not going well, you should be very critical of yourself. Find out what's necessary to improve things. All the time you should be thinking "What can I do to improve the standard of care for my patients, to improve the technique?"' (*Gynae*)

Technique and interaction with the patient go hand in hand. 'If there's more time to explain to the patient what's going on, and more time to help them through it, that adds to the satisfaction.' (*Gynae*)

Maintaining standards depends in the first place on the training, and in the second place on a process of self-evaluation.

In America, the evaluation process is more systematic, because of the huge fees paid to the surgeons. In Britain it is more haphazard and left up to the individual surgeon. 'What every consultant worth their salt should do is what I do in my hospital. Every three weeks we go through all the specimens removed in operations and discuss the reason they were removed. If there's a whole series of normal uteruses, then something is wrong somewhere. It helps us analyse the results and evaluate them. Not everybody does this but the better units do.' (*Gynae*)

A continuing dilemma in the medical profession is that the need to train medical students and the importance of acquiring practical experience, means that in the NHS there is no guarantee that you will be seen or operated on by the consultant whose unit you attend. This reinforces the patient's dependence on consultants and their standard of training. It also underlines the trust that we place in the 'expert's' hands.

'Looking at patients generally and patients that come and see me, they have that trust. I'm sure they wouldn't be able to tell whether I, my registrar or my houseman was Mr X. This trust is an amazing thing, I hope we discharge the trust in a reasonable way.' (*Gynae*)

The Nurse

'I have a different perspective on a patient than a doctor. Being a woman myself, with some experience of the world, I know a patient's problems.' (*Staff Nurse*)

The team of nurses – ward sister, qualified nurses, trainees and auxiliaries – are all responsible for the standard of care on the ward. Their role includes the physical tending of patients, providing emotional support; the relief of physical pain and mental anxiety. 'It's very important to show them as much affection as possible; holding their hand to and from theatre. At all ages they need so much reassuring.' (*Staff Nurse*)

The aftercare by nursing staff left a deep impression on the women we interviewed: 'I was in for seven days and the staff were marvellous.' (*Fiona*)

'They were excellent nurses. One step ahead of you most of the time. Very good encouraging you gently to get up.' (*Jean*)

At Sally's hospital she was assigned a nurse for the first three days after the operation. 'It's a bit like when you're in labour and you have a midwife who stays with you, and you put your trust in her. You are nervous and to have that one nurse with you all the time, builds your confidence. If you were pushed too quickly from nurse to nurse, you could get panicky and it would slow down the healing process and everything.'

'The nursing care was absolutely superb. It wasn't the SRNs, it was the SENs who were obviously given a patient or two to look after. I was throwing up all the time. Sick everywhere. I kept apologizing and her sweet smile was there and she said "I wish you'd stop saying you're sorry."' (*Angela*)

'I never got to the pain stage, really, I had a fantastic Staff Nurse, who anticipated everything right the way through. I had my medication before the pain really got going. She did everything for me, including washing and putting toothpaste on my toothbrush.' (*Sandra*)

Elaine, unlike the others, was isolated from the main ward and remembered 'a sort of guardian angel who came in the middle of the night. She was the only person who gave me something which was long, long overdue. She was a Matron checking round the whole hospital – obviously one of the old brigade, she looked in the side wards. She sticks out in my mind because she administered something that helped. If I ever catch up with her, I'll give her a big hug.'

On the whole, women were positive about their nursing care, although they were aware that much depended on the staff rota during their stay. A more general complaint was lack of information from them.

'They didn't enlighten you medically, which I disliked.' (*Jean*)

'There was no one around who could give me a proper explanation of what was happening to me, or reasons why I had to have something done to me. For me, everything was done by auxiliaries, nurses without professional qualifications, or students.' (*Jenny*)

'I found it very hard. The nurses never spoke about it – what had been done to me or anything like that.' (*Louise*)

Our Staff Nurse felt communication was very important: as a nursing team and also with the patients. She felt: 'Sometimes the uniform can be a barrier. I tell them my Christian name, which is very unprofessional, but it helps. It makes it possible for patients to ask questions.'

Whether it is the uniform, lack of qualified staff, or the changing rota system which prevents continuity, it does seem that information isn't as forthcoming as it could be.

'We should be prepared for patients to ask questions. The anxieties are expressed by young and old. We don't put ourselves out enough to explain things; I think we should.' (*Staff Nurse*)

The Patient

The fourth role in the drama belongs to the patient. 'Doctors need patients just as much as patients need doctors.' (*Gynae*)

'I'd like to see women in control of their own bodies, and retaining that control; not allow the medical mafioso to take the whole thing over.' (*Jenny*)

'It used to be a man's world – it still is really, but we do have a little bit of power. We can choose what we do with our bodies.' (*Staff Nurse*)

What does the role of 'patient' entail?

For some it means handing over total responsibility to the doctors' care and judgement. 'Many patients accept what the surgeon says in total trust, which is not a bad thing. It is left to the surgeon to decide which approach is the safest and within her/his technical competence. Whatever s/he says to you, you do it.' (*Gynae*)

'I believe what they tell you; accept that they know better than I do. If that's what's necessary, then do it.' (*Margaret*)

'I rather handed over the whole matter to the professionals. They would know what was best for me. I was quite happy to go along with whatever was suggested. As a nurse, I became a shrivelling heap whenever I saw a doctor.' (*Jenny*)

But for others the patient role is more active. They are not always happy simply to trust the expert. They want to ask questions and play a full part in decisions that affect their bodies. Many doctors are defensive about patients asking questions because they fear their authority will be undermined. Fortunately, others are more open to the value of consulting with the patient as much as possible.

Speaking up

Getting the best from your doctor is a delicate balance between acknowledging the other's experience and specialist knowledge, and at the same time having the confidence to ask for all the information you want and not to be pushed into a decision before you are ready.

It is quite usual for even the most forthright among us to be struck dumb when confronted with a medical expert. The environment alone is daunting; you may be rushed; other people may be present. Above all, we tend to be very vulnerable because the subject under discussion is so very personal.

In our anxiety we are unwilling to antagonize the consultant. We fear that if we get on the wrong side of them, they'll take it out on us in some way during the operation. 'I thought if I said I don't want the students round, the consultant's attitude would be different.' (*Carole*)

Although this fear is usually unfounded, it is powerful enough to make us bend over backwards not to be a nuisance. For this reason we don't ask the questions we want to ask. We don't persist if information is withheld. We don't ask for a second opinion (our right even in the NHS). We even comply with treatment we find uncomfortable, embarrassing and humiliating.

'If I had to have it done over again, I would forget my shyness. I would be more pushy and ask everything I was thinking about. I just sat there all the time – it's stupid really.' (*Carole*)

How can we learn to speak up more effectively without aggressively telling the doctors their job or meekly accepting everything and everyone that comes our way?

The principle is clear: 'Patients who don't understand what has been done to them concern me, as their recovery rate is longer. Those who do understand what has been done to them will recover much more quickly.' (*Gynae*)

It's likely that if you don't ask, no one will tell you anything. So how then can we enquire?

Be specific, and repeat your question until you get a satisfactory reply.

Sandra recommended taking the time to 'write down on a bit of paper everything that bothers you. When the doctor does the rounds, or you visit the consultant, you've got your questions ready to ask. You can do it again before leaving hospital because most patients are seen then. And the same when you visit your GP. Otherwise you'll forget. Most doctors won't mind.'

Another recommendation when seeing the consultant came from Sally: 'Take along a friend who makes no comments, but takes down what's being said. Otherwise you can come out and find you've forgotten something and then wish you'd asked something else.'

From personal experience we believe this to be an excellent idea, but wondered if it would just encourage the consultant's paranoia!

Our gynaecologist was quite in favour of a patient bringing someone along to the consultation and said he personally would encourage it although he admitted, 'Some doctors tend to resent third parties. But I think it's lovely that someone comes with them – a neighbour if they haven't got a spouse, or a relative. I think most people should encourage that and not find it difficult. It's *very, very* important and helps tremendously.'

Speaking up assertively is important, but it's only fair to note that sometimes this can be misinterpreted by doctors.

Sally was very disheartened in her attempt to keep a helpful diary of her symptoms, which was thoughtlessly discarded by her consultant. But she still recognized the need to be persistent. 'I found recently that you get more help if you have the attitude whereby you ask the questions and you don't tell them what you want and imply you know what's best for you. That comes down to confidence and I've not always been like that.'

Equally important is speaking up afterwards, if things go wrong or you want further information. We have already described the significance of the report back to the GP. Apart from it being personally important to express your feelings, it also means your report may benefit future patients.

Even if nothing has gone wrong, you may wish to know what has been removed. Astonishingly, this information will never be given automatically to the patient. It is assumed that the report is sent to the GP and s/he will eventually inform you of its contents Although in some countries patients who go from one specialist to the next carry their own comprehensive reports with them, in Britain we are dependent on our relationship with our GP for this information. Nevertheless, the gynaecologist agreed it was a reasonable request to make, although it wasn't normal procedure. 'If you asked for a report I would think you were making a fuss. If you took notes it would be better, although some doctors *hate* patients taking notes, they get quite paranoid.'

We cannot be sure of the correct approach to obtaining information, but we suggest you submit your questions with tact and diplomacy. You may find the following guidelines helpful:

- Bear in mind the doctor's paranoia.
- Make a list of areas you wish to discuss: fears, questions, anxieties.
- Don't wave the list threateningly or aggressively at the doctor or consultant.
- Explain that the list is intended purely to make the best possible use of her/his time, and to allay your concerns.
- If you can't take someone along, and you want to take notes, explain they are a memory prompt rather than notes to be used as evidence against them!

7
In Hospital

In this chapter we use the experiences and descriptions of the women we interviewed in combination with the experience of the gynaecologist and staff nurse, to give you a picture of what you can expect to happen during your hospital stay.

Each individual's experience is going to be slightly different, but we feel the range of events and circumstances and reactions recorded give a clear idea of how anyone anticipating hysterectomy might make the best of her stay.

The fourteen women in our sample stayed in hospitals around the country. Some went privately; some on the NHS. Their length of stay ranged from the shortest of six days to the longest, sixteen days, and anything in between.

Before the Operation

Arrival

'It is very important, the minute they walk in the door to make them feel welcome. Don't send them straight away to get undressed. Show them round first, give them a cup of tea, let them feel the environment before they become part of it.'

This is what our Staff Nurse said she and her colleagues tried to do, while admitting, 'We don't always get the time to do it.' Lack of time is probably the reason/excuse given by many hospitals for not being able to welcome patients coming in for major surgery, and for not putting us more at ease.

Going into hospital is bewildering and confusing. Not only because of the strangeness of the environment and because we are fearful about how the operation will go, but also because we have to be dependent on strangers for our lives. We must lose a sense of personal identity as we succumb to the role of 'patient'. We often feel helpless, simply because we do not know the routine: we don't know what to do when or how, without being told.

If you are a nurse yourself, you might think it would be much easier to enter into hospital routine. But as Jenny (a psychiatric nurse) described, in her situation she had to cross 'an invisible boundary between being nurse and patient'. Her fears were just those that any woman patient is likely to feel. 'It was a busy gynae unit. Although I had been in there before on a number of occasions, I still had the fears – they haven't told me to take my clothes off, so do I take them off? They haven't told me to get into bed, so do I get in or do I go to the day room?'

Even if you have been accompanied by your partner or a friend, there will inevitably come the time when they have to leave. This can be quite a low moment for many women. It would be an enormous boon if there could be a nurse or volunteer helper on hand at that particularly vulnerable time to help the patient settle in and answer all those worrying questions, as she makes the difficult transition from outsider to in-patient.

Taking the right things into hospital can also be helpful. The Staff Nurse warned against nylon nightwear, which becomes very uncomfortable in the warmth of the hospital ward, and recommended cotton nightwear. Sandra suggested a V-shaped orthopaedic pillow which she found extremely useful after the operation for support in bed. 'You put it behind you and it keeps you upright. Far more comfortable than the pillows continually sliding down.'

Routine preparation

Before your operation you will have various tests. Your blood-pressure and your pulse will be checked; a urine sample will be taken to check for infection or any irregularities; a sample of blood will be taken for analysis to match, in case you may need a blood transfusion; and sometimes the anaesthetist will visit you to check your chest and lungs.

'I was very much reassured by the anaesthetist's visit, because the anaesthetic was the thing I was most afraid of.' (*Nikki*)

Jean was similarly reassured. She was 'terrified of being over-anaesthetized and coming out a vegetable. You are more likely to die from the anaesthetist's mistake than from the surgeon's knife. I told the anaesthetist about my concern and about my always being sick afterwards. He said, "I'm glad you told me because we can give you an injection as soon as you come round, we won't wait for you to be sick. We'll give you a jab every half hour to stop your nausea."'

If you're lucky, you may get a visit from your surgeon before the operation, and if you're extremely lucky, a visit from your GP.

If you are admitted to a teaching hospital, be prepared for some of these routine tasks and interviews to be carried out by medical students. Students can appear at the foot of your bed without supervision, to take a case history or examine you. They must then write a report and present it on the consultant gynaecologist's ward round. This can be somewhat disconcerting and you may want to check out who they are if they don't say anything to you first. (As a patient you do have the right to refuse student examinations if you wish, even if you are in a teaching hospital.)

Jenny disliked the experience of being used as a 'teaching aid' without prior introduction. 'I felt like making a protest, when three students came to examine and interview me with no by-your-leave, no identification or explanation of who they were. I think they thought if they said they were medical students I would not have allowed them to touch me. In fact, once I knew they were part of my consultant's team, and what they were doing, I was happier.' Surely an introduction is nothing more than common courtesy, especially if you are about to conduct a vaginal examination!

What happens next, after the routine tests and administrative paperwork, will depend on how long you are admitted to hospital prior to your operation. You may go in twenty-four hours before, or the evening before an early morning operation. You will not be given anything to eat or drink twelve hours before the operation. It is likely that your pubic hair will be removed. This is never exactly a pleasure, but it is quite painless and fortunately nowadays, most of your hair is left intact; it is only considered necessary to remove a one-inch strip across the top and does not extend down to your genitals.

You'll be anxious to know what's going to happen next, but it is useful to ask the right people for information and not listen to idle gossip which may be misleading as well as frightening. 'Because you are in a gynae ward, there are generally other women who are at different stages of hysterectomy. The trouble is that discussion is pretty uninformed and often alarmist.' (*Jenny*)

'You have to keep your ears open. Some people pass on false information to others going down to theatre which could worry them. You have to be very watchful and careful.' (*Staff Nurse*)

'The night before my operation I was having my evening meal and someone asked me what I was in for. I replied "Just D and C and hysterectomy." An older woman overheard my conversation and said: "You mustn't let them do a D and C and hysterectomy on you. They only do that when you've got cancer." I knew that was a possibility but I had buried it away. I went back to my bed white. My neighbour in the ward said: "What the hell is the matter with you? You look as though you've seen a ghost!" Even though I wouldn't have admitted it at the time, I was very worried about cancer and the other patient's comments hadn't helped.' (*Jean*)

You may want to know what happens when you regain consciousness. 'They are told a drip and a catheter are both routine, so when they wake up they are not worried about it . . . Often they may be in a room alone when they wake up so that we can keep a special eye on them. They are warned about this so that when they wake up they don't feel "where am I? Perhaps something has gone wrong."' (*Staff Nurse*)

Unfortunately, not all nursing staff or indeed consultants see fit to pre-warn patients what to expect when waking up. This leads to some unpleasant and frightening surprises. Linda woke up 'horrified' to find herself connected to a drip. Carole, too, said it was 'horrible to find a tube inside' her abdomen with a pad on the outside to collect the blood.

Drips

A drip refers to an apparatus which feeds the patients by 'dripping' saline (a salt and sugar solution) from a container down the tube directly into a vein in the back of your hand.

After an anaesthetic you become dehydrated and thirsty, but you are not allowed to take any fluid by mouth for twenty-four hours – this drip stops you starving or drying out completely. A drip is not always attached and you may have a damp cloth passed over your lips to ease your thirst instead. The drip method is often used to stop you feeling too parched and to maintain the correct level of sodium (salt) in the blood.

In addition to the saline drip, some doctors nowadays prefer to combine this system with a second one which automatically pumps correct amounts of pain-killing drugs into your body in the same way. This would result in two or three thin tubes leading into the back of your hand instead of one, with perhaps the third for a blood transfusion should it be necessary.

Drains

The 'drain' refers to any method of draining off excess blood or tiny bits of tissue or debris left behind in the wound after surgery. In the case of hysterectomy there are two kinds of drain:

- A Readivac, which consists of a thin tube leading from the wound out into a bottle which can then be emptied when necessary.
- A Yates drain, which consists of a wad of sterile material acting as a sponge to absorb the blood and debris; it is replaced with a fresh wad of material as necessary.

Seeing the blood accumulate in the bottle or on the padding, does frighten many people, particularly if they are not expecting it. It is apparently quite simple to cover the drain so that it is out of sight, but for some obscure reason not all nursing staff bother. One woman we spoke to said she was so shocked to see the bottle of blood and debris that she asked the nurse to remove what she thought had been left behind by the previous occupant!

Catheter

A catheter is a thin narrow tube inserted through the vagina, up the urethra into the bladder to syphon off the urine when, for some reason like an operation, the bladder fails to function properly on its own. You will be catheterized automatically (tube inserted) while you are unconscious in theatre to ensure the bladder is empty before the operation begins. If you have a vaginal hysterectomy the catheter is likely to be left in for some time afterwards: twenty-four hours to five days.

Whether or not you are catheterized after an abdominal hysterectomy depends very much on the surgeon. Our gynaecologist explained that the catheter is used to prevent possible damage to the bladder. 'After the operation, patients have fluids which come down from the kidney and accumulate in the bladder. If the patient is under quite heavy sedation, she may not realize her bladder is full – neither does anyone else. No one comes to check and perhaps no one feels it because it's a sore spot. The ward system may mean that it is not checked until the following morning. During that time the bladder overdistends, you can't pass urine and they put in the catheter. However, because the bladder has become overstretched, it won't regain its normal muscle tone for five to ten days. The bladder may distend again and again. If the catheter is left in you can get infections in the catheter, which is very common; then you get cystitis so that not only does the bladder not function properly, it has become infected as well.'

The way to ensure these complications don't arise in the first place, is for the consultant to leave strict instructions to the ward sister and her staff, to make sure patients pass urine within six hours of the operation. If this cannot be done naturally, then it is best to put a catheter in, and take it out again once the bladder is empty. It all depends on the skill of the ward staff and the quality of post-operative care.

This covers most of the likely experiences involved in the lead up to your operation, as well as some of the things you might like to know in advance so that you are not taken by surprise when you come round. Now we come to the operation itself.

The Operation

What follows next is a 'stitch by stitch' account of what happens from the time you leave your bed in the ward, to the time you return having had your hysterectomy. It is an explicit account, so if you feel a bit squeamish, we advise you to skip the next few pages. On the other hand, reading it could allay many of your worst fears, and increase your knowledge of exactly what happens to your body after the anaesthetic takes over and you are in the hands of the operating staff – surgeons, anaesthetists and theatre nurses.

The surgery described applies to abdominal hysterectomies: for surgical method in vaginal hysterectomies, see pages 76-7.

Down to theatre

Your pre-operative medication (probably valium) will have been administered on the ward, and you will have changed from your nightdress into a plain gown. You may leave the ward/your room, in your own bed or on a special trolley. In any event, you will trundle down to theatre feeling drowsy.

On arrival in theatre reception, your name and diagnosis is checked, and the nature of the operation confirmed by a member of the theatre staff to ensure you have the correct operation for your complaint.

Due to staff shortages you may be left alone for a while – it is a distressing time and this practice should be condemned. A friendly face helps, so if you are not lucky enough to be introduced to a nurse who has been allocated to be with you throughout the operation, look out for the surgeon, perhaps the anaesthetist you saw the day before or, if you're really lucky, your own GP if s/he has turned up for the occasion.

Your medical notes are then handed to the theatre sister in charge that day, who will check you have had nothing to eat or drink recently, and whether you have false teeth, dental crowns or bridges or specific allergies to drugs.

The consent form is checked for your signature. (You probably did this the day before, fully conscious, before having had any medication).

Out for the count

The anaesthetist will give you an intravenous injection of anaesthetic, usually in one of the veins on the back of your hand. This sends you off to sleep before you can count to five. It paralyses you so that all your muscles are completely relaxed.

A small tube is inserted down your throat into the trachea. There is a small bag on the end of the tube which inflates inside the trachea, preventing oddments of food straying from the stomach into your lungs. If anything does float around, the bag stops secretions trickling into your lungs; when this happens bubbles appear and the anaesthetist sucks the problem away.

Hitched up for life

Next, you will be hitched-up to the life-support equipment: a machine which systematically pumps air and anaesthetic gasses into and out of your lungs, an electrocardiograph (ECG) machine, and a blood-pressure machine, so that all through the operation there is a complete picture on a paper trace print-out of your blood-pressure, pulse and heartbeat available to everyone in the theatre. Should there be the slightest deviation in the normal way your body functions, it is immediately brought to everyone's attention, and appropriate 'rescue' action taken to ensure your survival.

The 'inner sanctum'

It is now time to enter the inner sanctum of the operating theatre itself. You are completely limp – we hesitate to say a dead weight! You will be transferred from your own bed or trolley to the theatre operating table. (Back pain experienced by some people when they wake up is often attributed to bad handling at this point. It depends how strong and careful the porters are and how heavy you are, as to whether or not you are thumped or gently lowered onto the operating table.)

Once on the operating table, a nursing assistant will empty your bladder of urine with a catheter to make it easier for the surgeon to work inside the abdomen. Your vagina is painted with 'Bonney's Blue' antiseptic dye to cleanse and sterilize the area.

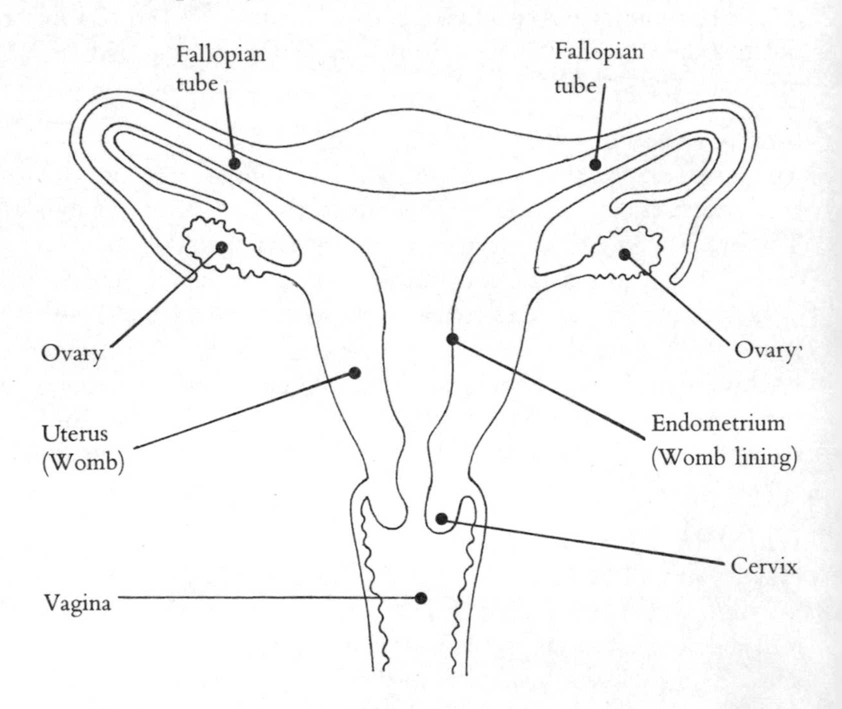

Diagram 2: Womb, Ovaries, Fallopian Tubes in Place Before Hysterectomy

Opening up

The skin is sterilized with iodine or a similar compound. Sterile drapes are hung over your body. Next, the surgeon makes the horizontal, bikini or vertical incision through the abdomen, and feels around inside. Your intestine and bowel are in the way, so you are tilted head down, in much the same way as you are often tipped backwards in a dentist's chair, and the force of gravity pulls the intestine and bowel out of the way, giving the surgeon room to manoeuvre and see what's going on more clearly.

A pack of sterile and moist towels is made up next, and one or two placed in the abdomen to keep the intestines to one side.

Clamps are then secured to the round ligament, Fallopian tubes and suspensory ligaments on either side of the uterus. These structures are then carefully cut and tied up neatly with cat gut or silk.

The uterus is pulled up, the bladder is pulled forward and a cut is made between the bladder and uterus, pushing the bladder out of the way.

More clamps are secured to the uterine arteries, making sure the ureters, which run close by, are not clamped as well. The uterine arteries are then cut and tied up.

With the exception of a sub-total hysterectomy where the cervix is retained, the cervix is then freed from the top of the vagina, which is then cut open so that the cervix is removed with the uterus.

Depending on the method of hysterectomy (see Diagrams 3a, b and c) the ovaries and Fallopian tubes may also be removed at this point. Once the uterus is taken out, it is examined carefully for anything untoward and unexpected. It is then passed to the pathologist for more detailed inspection in the laboratory later.

Next, the surgeon stitches the vagina closed at the top, ties up all the major pedicles, closes the peritoneum in the pelvis; s/he then checks the bowel, liver, spleen, stomach and colon to see if they, too, are healthy. It is at this stage the appendix is often removed if it looks unhealthy, to prevent trouble or the possibility of another operation.

Closing up

A careful check is made to ensure there is no bleeding from the delicate needlework so far completed. The peritoneal cavity and then the abdomen are closed with more stitches.

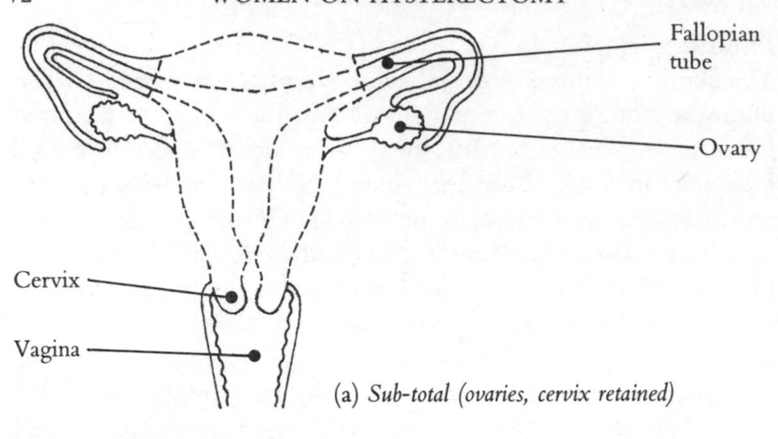

(a) *Sub-total (ovaries, cervix retained)*

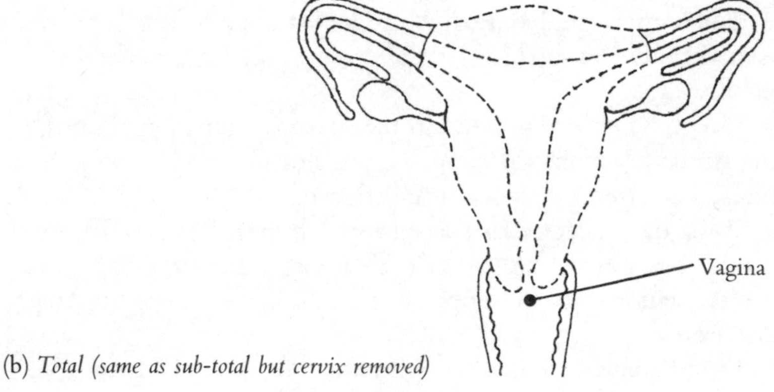

(b) *Total (same as sub-total but cervix removed)*

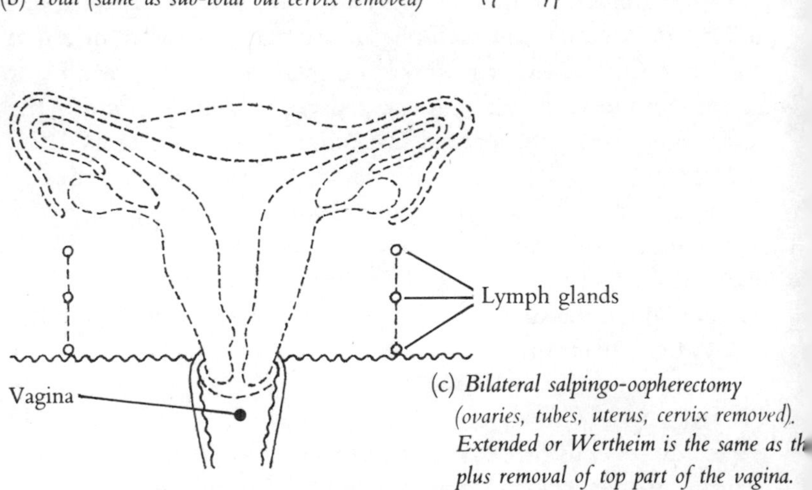

(c) *Bilateral salpingo-oopherectomy (ovaries, tubes, uterus, cervix removed). Extended or Wertheim is the same as th plus removal of top part of the vagina.*

Diagram 3: Parts of the Body Removed by Hysterectomy

During closure, the theatre sister in charge will check that the number of swabs and instruments used and removed, corresponds with the number previously counted and meticulously recorded on a special board in theatre, *before* the operation. The surgeon asks if the number of instruments and swabs tallies. If there is any doubt at all, everyone stops until there has been a re-count and all the equipment accounted for. If there is something missing (and it does happen), an X-ray machine is summoned and the patient is X-rayed, and the missing item discovered. It is then immediately removed.

As the surgeon closes the abdomen s/he might put in a small polythene drain tube. This is necessary because after all the dissection, stitching, and handling of bits and pieces, there is bound to be some capillary haemorrhage (slight bleeding). If it is drained off it cannot fester and cause unnecessary complications later on as you heal.

Complications in theatre

Another serious problem is deep vein thrombosis (DVT); this is when a blood clot forms in the vein of the leg and suddenly detaches itself, travels to the heart and then the lungs, where it can block the blood flow. In order to prevent blood clotting, some patients at risk are given prophylactic anti-coagulants to dissolve the blood clot, or perhaps put in specially designed boots with a pump that squeezes the calves, pumping blood round the body. Alternatively, patients are put in special stockings, or the surgeon goes to the foot of the operating table, lifts up the leg and manipulates the ankles or calves.

All sewn up

Once all the cut and frayed parts of your body are sewn up carefully and neatly, the anaesthetic is reversed. You start to breathe under your own steam without the help of machinery. As that happens, the tube in your throat is removed, and you begin to breathe normally, perhaps coughing a little. Your throat may be sore when you regain consciousness.

You will be whisked to the recovery room, and given something to alleviate the pain immediately. A nurse will supervise your recovery until you are fully conscious.

Anaesthetic drugs have a peculiar effect on most of us. It is now that we are most likely to divulge our innermost, uncontrollable thoughts and secrets. But don't worry, the nurses are sworn to secrecy and are the soul of discretion!

Back to your bed

From the recovery room you will be taken back to your own bed on the ward.

The whole process takes little more than an hour from the time you leave the ward until the minute you return. The time taken depends on the skill and care of the surgeon. A good one will take forty minutes to complete a hysterectomy. But speed is not always the sign of a good surgeon; the faster they are, the less likely they are to make essential after-checks such as for internal bleeding.

The safety net

You may wonder why operations cost so much; it is due to the number of people indirectly or directly responsible for your care while you are in the operating theatre.

Porters, nurses, perhaps a couple of post-graduate student gynaecologists assisting or observing; the consultant surgeon, a first assistant or registrar, one or two anaesthetists and perhaps a special anaesthetic nurse, are all in attendance. Each and every one of them focusing on *you* and what's happening to your body.

It could be a somewhat daunting prospect or a tremendous comfort to know so many people are there specifically to see you through the ordeal safely.

Choosing the Right Hysterectomy

In most cultures a woman's self image relies heavily on how she and others view her body.

Unfortunately, unless we are fortunate enough to stumble across a sympathetic surgeon who is sensitive to our feelings about being scarred, we are seldom invited to discuss our thoughts on the subject of which type of hysterectomy and scar we would prefer, given the particular circumstances surrounding the need for the operation. Ultimately the final decision is left to the surgeon.

The primary factors that dictate the method of hysterectomy are:

- the condition of the cervix, uterus, ovaries, *and*
- the individual preference of the surgeon chosen (usually by your GP) to carry out the operation.

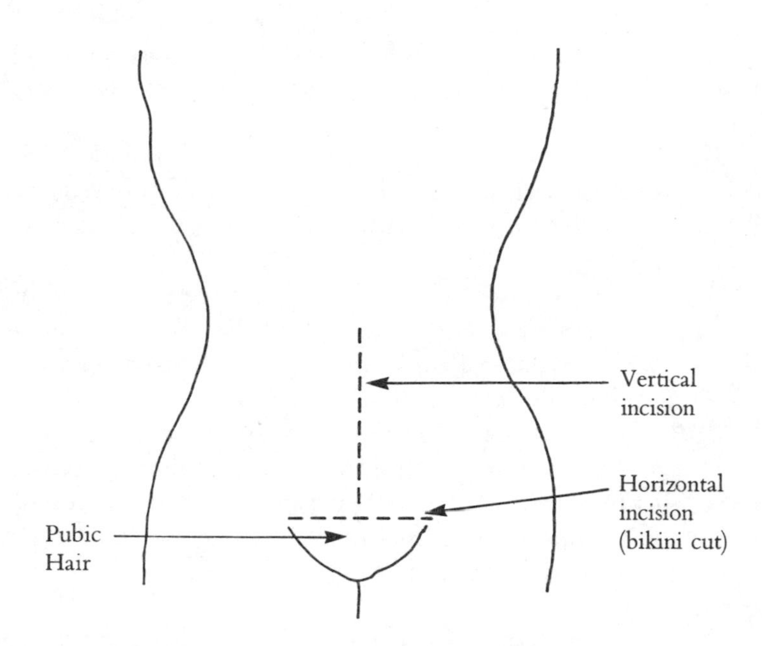

Diagram 4: Abdominal Hysterectomy – incision approximately 6-8 inches (15-20cm)

They'll do it their way

Each surgeon operates and cares for patients differently. For the very important vessels – uterine arteries/ovarian pedicles – some surgeons use cat-gut stitches which dissolve as the body heals; others use linen or silk, or some other non-absorbable compounds.

Some surgeons use metal clips to pull the abdominal skin together. These can be painful when removed and are unsightly; others put a linen or silk stitch underneath the skin so there is nothing visible at all except a couple of little beads at either end. These can be painlessly removed.

Some surgeons always catheterize their patients for a few days after the operation; others leave strict instructions with nursing staff to ensure the bladder is emptied six to twelve hours after the operation either naturally or, if this is too painful, by catheterization.

Some surgeons arrange for a painkiller to be administered 'magically' when it is most needed, via an intravenous drip; others prescribe four-hourly painkilling injections into your buttocks.

Sub-total hysterectomy

The easiest type of hysterectomy from the surgeon's point of view and the one from which patients recover most rapidly is the 'sub-total hysterectomy': cervix and ovaries and Fallopian tubes are left intact.

Sadly, since the cervix is now recognized as a possible cancer site, its removal is automatic unless: (a) you specifically request it to be left in place, (b) it is healthy, *and* (c) the surgeon agrees to your request.

'There was a time when we didn't remove the cervix and then patients developed carcinoma [cancer] of the cervix so then we felt we ought to remove it automatically. But if a patient expresses the wish to have her cervix retained, and provided she agrees to come for cervical smears annually, then I see no reason why the cervix shouldn't be retained. It's just a little unorthodox.' (*Gynae*)

Leaving the cervix intact makes it much easier for the surgeon because it is unnecessary to first cut into and then stitch the top of the vagina, and consequently avoids the delicate and accident-prone ureter.

However, in spite of all this, sub-total hysterectomy is pronounced 'a thing of the past'.

Are cervical smear tests required after hysterectomy?

'After the op I asked if I needed cervical smears – do I still have my cervix, and he looked it up and said don't bother.' (*Elaine*)

'If the cervix has been removed you can forget about it, unless the hysterectomy was done for malignant disease: there might still be cancer in the residue of the vagina, so you should go back for a couple of repeat smear tests. If they prove negative, that's all right, you needn't have any more.' (*Gynae*)

'There are different views on this. Some surgeons see patients for ever. If the patient is receiving radiotherapy, it interferes very greatly in the interpretation of the smear test so that it is of no value. It varies from case to case.' (*Gynae*)

Vaginal hysterectomy

Technically, this is the most difficult hysterectomy. Generally speaking, most surgeons avoid vaginal hysterectomy unless the uterus has dropped (prolapse – see Chapter 3) which makes it easy. Of course, some surgeons are wizards at this operation and always do hysterectomy vaginally. But most surgeons are deterred by the complications that may arise following the removal of the uterus via the vagina unless there is a prolapse.

If the womb is to be removed through the vagina, the surgeon proceeds in much the same way as for abdominal hysterectomy, but this time s/he sits in front of your open legs and makes the necessary incisions up through the top of the vagina, instead of down through the abdomen.

Not only is it technically very difficult to take the uterus out this way, demanding greater surgical skill, but undetected internal haemorrhaging at the time of the operation or immediately afterwards, could result in serious infection, and severe bowel problems, and even death.

The great advantage of vaginal hysterectomy is the absence of a scar and the more rapid recovery rate.

Complications after the operation

Serious complications resulting from a hysterectomy are rare. However, our consultant told us that amongst professionals there is an 'acceptable complication rate'. 'Even the best surgeons', he said, 'have complications.' They are due to:

- something unforeseen:
  1. tumour larger or more extensive;
  2. difficulty with stopping haemorrhage; patience and skill are needed. Surgeon should not feel s/he is under pressure to complete the operation because another case or emergency is waiting;
  3. anaesthetic complications, e.g., allergies;
  4. previous unknown heart complications.
- Trauma to other structures during a complex dissection. (Excessive rummaging around and handling or accidental cutting of organs close to the uterus – bladder, ureter, bowel and rectum.)
- So much depends on:
  1. pre-operative assessment – history, examination, investigation.

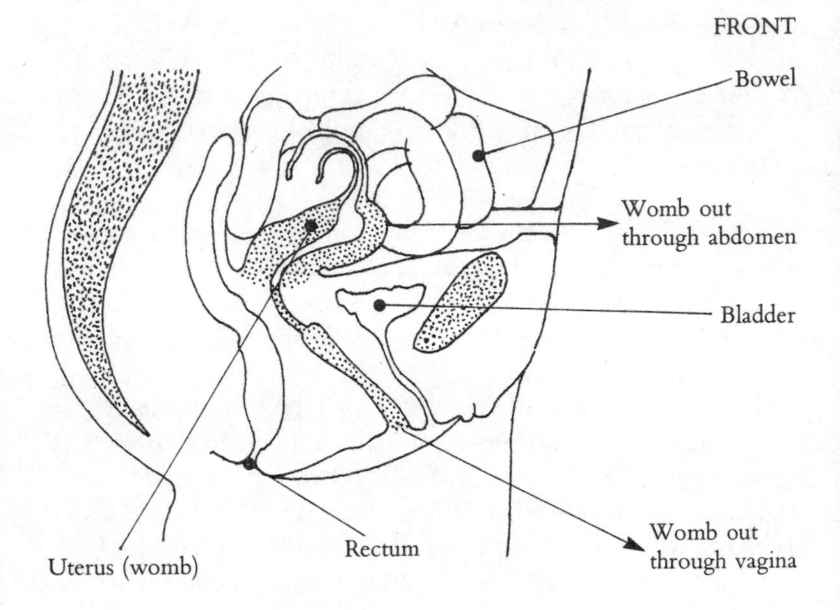

Diagram 5a: Before Hysterectomy

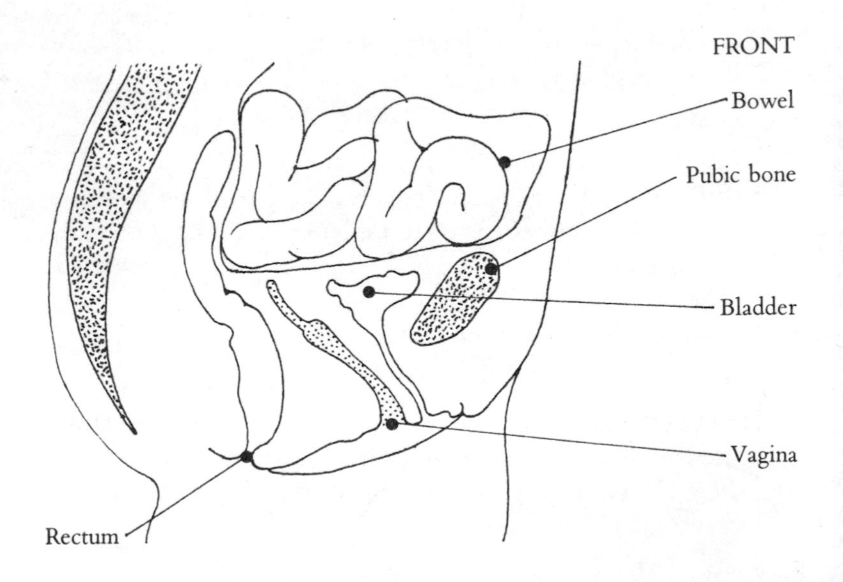

Diagram 5b: After Hysterectomy

2. Skill of the surgeon and anaesthetist.
3. Calm, efficient, unhurried atmosphere in theatre.

On average one patient in every 1000 will suffer ureteric damage, and one patient in 500 will suffer bladder damage. Damage to the bowel and rectum is much rarer.

It is important to remember that, although complications may arise after your operation, once detected, they can be quickly and safely rectified.

Ureteric damage: occurs because the most difficult part of a hysterectomy is clamping the uterine artery in exactly the right place, and *not* clamping the ureter by mistake. Damage to the ureter is the biggest problem. It is rare but it does occur. The surgeon may not realize it at the time and the first time it becomes apparent that something is wrong is, afterwards, when the patient complains of loin pains or leaks urine from the vagina. As long as the surgeon recognizes and takes heed of the symptoms, and knows what has happened and what to do, it is easily remedied. Another operation implanting the ureter into the bladder quickly solves the problem.

Damage to the bladder: is another complication. An opening/hole appears between the bladder and the vagina and urine leaks into the vagina. This hole usually closes naturally in six weeks, but if it does not, another operation is needed.

Ileus: describes the disturbance of the bowel that everyone will experience to some degree. After any operation the bowel shuts down for twelve to thirty-six hours. This is why patients have all their fluids and food intravenously until 'ileus has passed', in other words, the normal peristaltic motion of the bowel has recommenced and the rectum is able to empty again.

Complex dissection: a Wertheim hysterectomy has a higher mortality rate according to our consultant. 'A quarter of one per cent, because there is so much work to do. Risk of haemorrhage is much greater. One study showed that eighteen per cent of patients who have Wertheim hysterectomy suffer permanent urinary disabilities due to ureteric damage. Post-operative recovery from Wertheim hysterectomy is also slower. But against all this should be balanced the unpleasantness and hazards of radiotherapy. The patient would die without radical surgery to remove the disease.

But if you are alive, a degree of disability is a small price to pay.' (*Gynae*)

After the Operation

Coming round

Coming round after the operation, we enter a twilight phase, where intermittent moments of consciousness and an awareness of coming through an ordeal are shrouded in a general feeling of being cocooned against the outside world.

Although we are heavily sedated, it is an important time because, temporarily, we are not inhabiting our bodies, and until we regain full consciousness and control, we are vulnerable. For this reason it can be a tremendous comfort to have your partner, a close friend or relative with you while you come round, until you feel more fully in charge of yourself. Obviously, you won't be able to speak to that person – it's just the fact that there's a caring presence near you which matters. You gradually become more aware of your surroundings.

'Although the nursing staff were bewildered by my friend's silent vigil, it made all the difference to me as I floated backwards and forwards between consciousness.' (*Nikki*)

Although memories of this time will be blurred and hazy, one thing the women all remembered was passing water for the first time.

Jenny was the only one who woke up with a catheter in place. This had been inserted in theatre. 'It's uncomfortable to have in. I felt as though I was peeing all the time. It was terribly tight in the urethra. I was more troubled by the catheter than by almost anything else.'

Margaret was catheterized one day after her operation. 'I did pass urine, but not enough for the nurses. The next day they decided I still hadn't done enough. They put a catheter up and it poured away. It didn't hurt having the catheter at all. They put a tube up, the urine drained down and out. I just had it that one time.'

For other women the mere threat of a catheter, either having experienced it before or after childbirth, or simply from reputation, proved to be quite a motivation to pass water through their own efforts! 'I had read how awful it could be to be catheterized. It was fear of the unknown, so when they said we'll give you a few more hours and then . . . I thought, "Right, I'm not having that." I didn't want to be messed about with again.' (*Sally*)

Fiona was keen not to have a catheter because she associated catheters with patients suffering from bladder infection. 'They said to me, "See if you can do without a catheter, really do try and get out of bed." It took me an hour, but I got out. They helped me sit on a commode; left me there until I went. I thought I was never going to pass water, but eventually I did. It was a marvellous relief.'

It was as well Angela managed on her own because she said at the interview, 'I would have left, had I known about the possibility of being catheterized.'

Jean showed remarkable persistence, as did the nurses taking care of her: 'I thought, "I must spend a penny, because if I don't, knowing my luck, they'll catheterize me tomorrow like when you have a baby." So I asked for a commode and they got me out of bed. Of course, I didn't really want to go, but mentally I *did* want to go. They were very patient, they lifted me into a sitting position and then on to the floor and then they held me and said, "take your feet off the ground and we'll sit you down." They ran all the taps in the ward and nothing happened. I sat on the loo surrounded by my jars. After eleven flushes, I emptied my bladder a little bit at a time. Flush, spent a little bit, waited for it to refill, flush again. They said, "have you got it down to ten yet, because we're running out of water!"'

Nikki was impressed by the ingenuity of the nursing staff's patient attempts to get her to empty her bladder. 'After the bedpan, running the taps in the bathroom and the basin, the final touch was slowing trickling warm water down over my genitals and *bingo*!'

As the Staff Nurse said: 'It's very important that they pass urine. That's a trick. They do eventually . . . we never give up.'

Moving about at last

Whatever the method of hysterectomy, particularly after abdominal surgery, one of the inevitable hurdles to face and overcome is how to move around.

Jean was worried about her stitches 'pinging and splitting open', but her neighbour helped. 'I was fortunate in that I was next to someone who had had her hysterectomy one week before me. I looked at her and thought, "If you can get in and out of bed after a week, I will." She told me things like if you come back from theatre lying down, don't think you'll split open when you stand up.'

You may be attached to cumbersome drip tubes and you may have no idea how to sit up or get out of bed without doing yourself any damage.

'For about forty-eight hours we keep them sedated; nice and quiet until we get them sitting up and taking fluids. When we tell them this, they can't believe it. The next day is the stage of making them feel comfortable. They are still quite sleepy. We don't keep them up long – half an hour or an hour. Some patients feel more comfortable in a chair. If that's where they are comfortable, that's where they stay. It's entirely up to them.' (*Staff Nurse*)

The importance of regaining mobility as soon as possible is to get your blood circulating normally. As Sally was advised, 'Deep breathing, moving your feet about a lot; keeping your legs and feet moving all the time to avoid blood clots.' Sally was lucky in that she was told by one of the nurses how to move. 'Getting in and out of bed was very cleverly put. Easy to get out but not so easy to get in again. I rolled to my right side and pushed up on my elbow.'

It is very important to move around but sometimes we can be a little over-enthusiastic. 'Three days after my operation I thought, "If they won't let me have a bath, I'm going to wash my feet." I was so pleased that I got my foot up into the washbasin; and they were so cross with me!' (*Jean*)

'I was up that same evening as if I hadn't had it done. They warned me, "You've got to take it easy." I think I tried to do too much because I felt so well. I couldn't believe I felt so little pain considering the surgery I'd had done. Three days later I couldn't move. I think it was delayed reaction.' (*Sally*)

Jean learned various techniques from the patient next to her. 'I'd like to have known at the time how to roll over in bed, how to get in and out and how to pull yourself up. The girl next door showed me how to roll the sheet into a ball, hang on to it and pull yourself up using it as a lever. I thought how easy it would be to tie a rope on the bed. Then you could use it to pull yourself up and pay it out to let yourself down again.'

It is important to remember that simple movements we

normally wouldn't think twice about, take on a huge significance after a major operation. Getting in and out of bed, turning over in bed, sitting up in bed and sleeping can be painful, so we often approach each movement with great caution. Most women interviewed were not shown any of these movements, apart from Sally, who was given clear instructions, and Louise who was also lucky: 'A very nice night nurse showed me how to sleep on my side, with a pillow. You lay half on the pillow with your stomach resting on it. I found that very comfortable, especially good if you can't sleep on your back.'

Simple, comfortable ways to get out of bed from a lying position are:

- In slow motion, bend your knees upwards;
- Keep your knees bent together and roll to your side;
- Swing your legs down over the edge of the bed;
- Sit up, pushing against the bed with your elbow of one arm and the hand of the other.
- To lie back down, reverse the steps.

It would be a good idea to practise this *before* you go into hospital so that you can get the hang of it.

Sustenance and nourishment

The normal sequence after surgery is a gradual intake of fluids *before* going on to solid food. Bodily systems have to get going again after their temporary shut-down under anaesthetic. As well as improving blood circulation, moving around will progress food through your intestines. It is helped by the wave-like (peristaltic) motion of the intestinal wall.

Under anaesthetic this natural motion stops, and it is very important that it is re-started as quickly as possible. Moving around helps, but we are unable to cope with solid food until the digestive system gets back to normal. That's why we are kept on a diet of fluids for the first day. You may be given fluids through the drip in your arm and, towards the end of the first twenty-four hours following the operation, be given a cup of tea. The first time you get something to drink will be at the discretion of the nursing staff who will first have checked for gurglings in your stomach, which indicates your bowel is on the move again.

You may feel thirsty when you come round, but you are

unlikely to feel hungry. Sometimes even a cup of tea can make you feel sick until your system settles down and begins to function normally. It is very common to feel nauseous after an operation; if there is danger that you will vomit, you will be given an anti-nausea injection.

Jean and Angela suffered vomiting attacks. They both had a history of reacting in this way to anaesthetics and warned the medical staff before the operation, but this didn't prevent problems arising. Jean and Angela felt the food given to them when they came round was quite inappropriate, given their condition.

Angela said: 'They just assume you can eat what's put before you – meat and two veg immediately.' For her, the trauma involved in trying to eat and then vomiting was the worst part of her whole hysterectomy experience. 'By the time I had been in hospital a week, I had lost a stone. It has taken me four years to reach the weight I was before I went in.'

Jean didn't want to eat at all after the anaesthetic because she knew it would make her sick. 'The nursing staff wouldn't have that, and tried to make me eat. I kept bringing it up. I remember on the third day, they got really cross and made me eat a cheese sandwich. I remember crying and saying, "For God's sake, it's bad enough having a belly-ache, without having a headache as well."'

The nausea is often caused by a reaction between the premedication drug and the anaesthetic. The pre-medication injection is administered to subdue patients on their way to theatre, but is not essential. If you react badly to anaesthetics, it might be worth discussing the possibility of foregoing the pre-medication, and thus avoid the inevitable consequences later.

On Sally's ward there was 'confusion about the right time to start eating solid food. Every surgeon had a different idea about when to start eating solids.'

Carole didn't feel like eating either and had a poor appetite. 'I was frightened to eat at first. I thought if I ate too much I would burst open so I didn't eat at all in hospital [six days].'

Elaine specifically remembered being given broad beans and baked beans, which highlights the irony that many hospitals seem to overlook the advice they give to patients to follow when they get home: follow a diet which will avoid constipation.

Wind

This can surely be counted as the most universal experience amongst the women interviewed, and one with which they could readily and painfully identify.

Many of the women were constipated, which is a predictable symptom after major surgery for the reasons described already. Unfortunately, because the bowel is temporarily blocked (it is quite normal not to empty it for seventy-two hours following the operation), gases build up inside the intestines and cannot escape because everything is not yet functioning properly.

It is difficult to talk about wind, and its passing, without some amusement. But it also happens to be extremely painful, and stands out as a particularly dreadful experience.

'It was most painful when I was constipated. I had never been constipated in my life before. Everyone had the most terrible wind. That was a great laugh. I was told when I first went in, the worst thing about this is the wind. The nurses said, "it will cause terrible agony and you'll think you're dying, but it's only wind." It wasn't only back passage wind, it was vaginal wind – even more embarrassing because you can't control it. I had terrible pressure on my tail. I felt as if everything had fallen down into my bottom – it was awful. They gave me some green stuff which shifted it eventually.' (*Fiona*)

Jenny reported 'awful constipation and wind'. Celia and Elaine said the wind was 'terrible'; Carole considered 'wind definitely the worst part'.

It came as a nasty shock to Sally. 'I came back so happy and relieved it was all over, until the wind set in on the third or fourth day . . . why didn't they *say* anything about the wind?' When the physiotherapist came round Sally asked about the pain and was prescribed different exercises to do.

Louise, too, was given some advice: 'I got warned as soon as I got in. The other girls said, "the wind is absolutely excruciating, drink plenty of Lucozade topped up with soda water; anything that will make you belch." It was terrible – I was in absolute agony. You'd get rid of it for a while, then it would come back. I was getting through bottles and bottles a day. But I was thankful they had warned me. It was one of the worst things besides the injections.'

'Some patients double up in pain – crying.' (*Staff Nurse*) It seems that some constipation and wind cannot be avoided, although not everyone suffered too badly. But it helps to be forewarned. The nurses will often administer a 'wind cocktail' upon request, which helps to relieve the symptoms but 'the best remedy for wind is a walk round the bed: it gets it moving much quicker than any medicine.' (*Staff Nurse*)

Pain

Pain is never welcome and is often frightening. Whatever the individual experience in hospital, everyone is bound to suffer pain at some time. 'I think we have to realize it can be pretty horrible afterwards, but then all operations are horrible afterwards. You won't go in and come out without some sort of pain. I think a lot depends on your pain threshold. Some people hit their little finger and carry on as if nothing has happened; others scratch themselves and are in dreadful agony for weeks.' (*Sandra*)

Our intention in explaining what you *might* find painful is not to cause undue alarm. Pain is often worse when it is unexpected, because then we are also frightened by not knowing how long it will last, and whether the pain means that something is wrong.

Before we look at what you may find painful, it is important to realize that there is always a limit to that pain. It won't persist for ever. Acute pain often disappears within a few days, and you will be off painkilling drugs well before leaving hospital.

Painkilling injections are always available, on request, or automatically for the first twenty-four hours. For some, this is the most painful time. Jean felt as though she had been jumped on and branded. 'I expected there to be an ache but it felt as if I had been burned. Even though I had had operations before, I had never experienced that sort of pain. It was as though someone had passed a burned knife right across my stomach; it was that continual burning sensation, rather than the aches and bruising, that was the worst. I had painkilling drugs in effervescent and injection form immediately afterwards, and Paracetamol for the last few days. I remember wanting them. Once you're in that situation your fear of drugs goes, and I thought "if I can have a painkiller and it enables me to walk around and sit up in bed, I'll have the painkiller." The same with sleeping tablets. Not when I came home – I didn't need painkillers by the time I came home [eight days].'

Sally tried to do without. 'I wanted to be alert, so after a day I refused the injections because they made me feel woozy. I thought I'd be clever and didn't have one all afternoon and evening. But by the time they came round with the drugs I got more and more agitated. I panicked as I was in so much pain. I then had sleeping pills and four Paracetamols a day while I was in hospital [ten days].'

Healing and holding it all together

There are no external stitches or scar in a vaginal hysterectomy. In abdominal hysterectomy the wound is closed up and held together with stitches or clips, so that the tissue can heal inside. If the skin isn't clipped together it is sewn up with a continuous thread of silk or cat gut and secured at either end with a tiny white plastic bead.

Only Carole described having clips. At first she wasn't aware of too much pain. It only hurt when she coughed and sneezed and it pulled on the clips. Her most painful experience was when they were removed. 'There was a nurse being examined for a test. She had never taken clips out in her life before . . . it took *half an hour* to remove the clips. It was a hot summer and she was nervous. In the end the sister in charge had to do it, they were so deeply embedded. When it was over she said, "Do you smoke?" I said, "no." "Well," she said, "you certainly deserve a good cup of tea after that." It was so very painful.'

If a wound drain has been inserted, as described on page 67, its removal may be painful. It depends on which kind of drain it is (Readivac or Yates), how long it has been there and how it is taken out.

If the drain is removed a couple of days after the operation, it will be much less painful than if it is left for longer and your tissue has a chance to heal round it. Carole found it very 'painful' as they pulled it out. For Fiona: 'The worst pain was when they removed the drain because I had healed right over it. I heal very quickly. I screamed because they were pulling flesh. It was absolute agony. They were really cross with me. I don't know why they didn't understand that it was so painful. Two holding me down and one pulling it out. When they removed it I was shaking for three hours afterwards, a complete jibbering mess. At visiting time I was still shaking. My husband said, "My God, what have they done to you? It's four days after your operation and you're worse than when you came in." It's strange they don't realize why . . .' It *is* strange that some nurses do not seem to understand that it can be very painful.

Jenny expected to have pain but didn't. When they removed her wound drain 'it felt very cold. It seemed to go on forever and made me feel slightly sick. It was smooth and slithery coming out.'

When the time comes to have the stitches, clips or drain removed, you may want to have someone with you to hold your hand. Ask the Staff Nurse when they anticipate removing these items, so you can arrange for it to coincide with a visit perhaps from a close friend or partner.

'I had anticipated someone being around for the removal of the stitches because I thought that would be painful. In fact, it was the drain that proved to be absolutely ghastly, particularly as I wasn't expecting it to be at all painful. I just screamed and screamed for half an hour as they pulled and pulled. It was only afterwards I realized that as I heal quickly, they were pulling against the tissue which, after four days, had begun to heal round the drain tube.' (*Nikki*)

In fact, none of the women interviewed recalled removal of the stitches being painful. Exactly when these external stitches are removed will depend on the surgeon's preference. It could be any time between five and ten days after the operation, or just before you leave hospital.

Friendly support

Because of the unfamiliarity of being in hospital and the various ups and downs you go through, the help of other patients and the nursing care received can make a great difference to your progress.

In Carole's hospital, she found that 'once the operation was over, you were just a number. No-one had time for you or helped you. You get all the attention when you first go in; you have what you go in for, and that's it – you've got to look after yourself after that.'

Other patients can be an important source of comfort. 'I always thought I was very shy. I don't like people seeing me at my worst. But when you are all in the same boat you can support each other.' (*Sally*)

Jean valued the reassurance given her by the girl in the next bed: 'Maybe they deliberately put me next to her because she was a week ahead and I could see the light at the end of the tunnel.'

Louise also valued the companionship, but still felt the odd one out, she felt "very young [thirty] compared to everyone else.'

From the perspective of either fellow-patients or nursing care, Elaine's experience certainly hit rock bottom. Her hospital stay was: 'A chapter of disasters from beginning go end'. Once they discovered her husband was a doctor, she was transferred from the main ward to a side ward on her own. Although this may have been intended as special treatment, it backfired: 'I was completely forgotten. The door was shut and there was no bell. The mattress was uncomfortable, it had old-fashioned buttons and I was sitting on the buttons but couldn't move. The back rest fell down, and I couldn't attract anyone's attention because there was no bell or buzzer. I was forgotten on the drug round, the tea round, and the surgeon even forgot to come and check me.' As a result, she had insufficient painkillers when she needed them because she couldn't communicate with the outside world. The only good thing about the room was that it opened directly on to the car park through French windows, so she had all the visitors she wanted. It's a pity no one thought to point out her predicament to one of the staff.

Post-op blues

On the third and fifth day after the anaesthetic, most women suffer from post-operative 'blues'. 'You can always tell what day it is when the tears start to come for no reason at all. They can't say what they're crying about. It's just routine. Sometimes it can be when they are ready to leave the hospital. It's not a particular type of person, it happens to any woman.' (*Staff Nurse*)

In Jenny's nursing experience she said, 'It is often more prevalent on a gynae ward than other surgical wards.' And the Staff Nurse said that it tended to happen 'more with women who have hysterectomies than other gynaecological operations.' Nobody can really say why this is so. The staff nurse suggested it could be relief that the operation is over and that we have survived, or possibly delayed shock. Jenny felt it could coincide with the withdrawal of intense physical care: 'You are unlikely to have a drip or drain by that time, and having become pretty institutionalized, having very close attention, very close care, it feels suddenly withdrawn.'

It's a time when 'you know you're are on your own and you've got to pick up . . . and most people do.' (*Sally*); it's a time when you can feel 'utterly desolate'. (*Jenny*); it's a time when you need 'lots of cuddles, lots of reassuring and a bit of a fuss'. (*Staff Nurse*)

Visitors

You'll probably find that hospitals allow one visitor only on the day of the operation – and it is usually the partner or a close relative that's expected.

The nurses are aware that it is important for many women to look good whatever the situation; so they encourage you to 'use your own smellies, have your hair combed and put on a bit of make-up. Having your own things around you, flowers, cards, contributes a great deal to the healing process.' (*Staff Nurse*)

Although visitors can be fun, our Staff Nurse cautioned against overloading. She felt that if the number exceeded two per patient it was too exhausting and 'patients just look drained, surrounded by chocolates and flowers. Those with large families find it particularly tiring. Sometimes you have to fight your way through to see the patient herself. I think it's too much.' She takes it upon herself to suggest discreetly that people leave, because the patient is never in a position to complain for herself: although she may be tired she does not want to offend those who have taken the trouble to visit.

A Summary of the First Five Days

The Staff Nurse gave her account of the first five days following a hysterectomy:

'We collect patients from theatre. Everything is made ready on the ward; drip stand, all the papers we are going to need. We try to keep the room nice and warm.

'The minute they come back, we put them into bed. First we check to see if there is any bleeding before covering them up. We check the sterile packs put inside the vagina for twenty-four hours to stop haemorrhage.

'Straightaway the patient is put on to half-hourly observation. We watch blood-pressure, pulse and blood-loss from the vagina. Painkilling injections are administered immediately so that patients suffer no pain or discomfort. They are usually given something four-hourly, automatically without being asked, to prevent nausea as well.

'They will be monitored half-hourly right through the first day. The night staff keep it up until they feel they can reduce it to one-hourly observation, and then four-hourly.

'When patients begin to come round, we reassure them that they are back, awake, and the operation has been successful.'

Day 2:
'They have a nice blanket bath and put on their own nightie again. It's very important that they pass urine. [Vaginal hysterectomies will have been catheterized already in theatre.]

'Some patients are reluctant to get out of bed, but it's important to get up to prevent chest infections and thrombosis. It's very important to be mobile as soon as possible. They will be seen by the doctor that morning, who will listen for bowel sounds. If they rumble away, they can have sips of water. By lunch-time if they tolerate sips of water, they can have some ice-cream and a cup of tea. If they tolerate that, by about 4 o'clock that afternoon we take down the drip, which keeps the vein open and makes sure they don't become dehydrated. They have ice cream because it's light, cool, no chewing and just slides down. Supper that day, they'll have some soup and a pudding if they want it. Again, it is something very light – trifle, jelly. If that all goes according to plan, that's a good start.'

Day 3:
'They can have either a bath or a strip wash and the dressing is removed. A check is made for blood loss in the vagina and the abdominal wound. Still on four-hourly observation. They now have a light diet: cornflakes, light lunch. Walk about, do what they want to do. They are still in their own quiet room, but if they want to, they can go down to the day room. We encourage them to go to the dining room for their meals; it's much better than sitting in their room moping, they can sit and talk with other patients. This is the day they are usually given suppositories to open the bowel.'

Day 4/Day 5:
'Stitches come out and from then on it's plain sailing with a few ups and downs – haematomas, constipation, but the majority of women sail through.

'Patients may stay fourteen days but most go home within ten to twelve days. Vaginal hysterectomies are mobile in forty-eight hours and may go home after a week.'

Preparing to Leave Hospital

Most women will have a clear idea of how long they will stay in hospital, well in advance of being admitted; anything from six to sixteen days. Sally had the unfortunate experience of being told to leave earlier than she expected, because she healed more quickly than anticipated. It wasn't so much the earlier departure date that upset her, it was being told one morning that she had to leave at midday that same day.

Things that may go wrong

Ideally, you will be in hospital until your wound is fully healed on the outside so that the internal healing can continue during convalescence.

A serious obstacle to healing is when the wound becomes infected. This can happen if a patient has an infection somewhere else in her body: for example, a carbuncle or a sore throat. Elderly, overweight, anaemic and diabetic patients are more prone to infection. Infection can also occur from something not properly sterilized in theatre; it can become infected through a drain being used and also through the surgeon's lack of care and competence, or entirely by chance.

For example, complications can be caused by failure to check that internal bleeding has stopped. A blood clot (haematoma) may form in the wound and this in turn may be infected by passing germs forming an abcess, which discharges into the wound. If this happens to you, it may take several weeks for the wound to heal.

So-called 'minor' complications after the operation were experienced by half the women we interviewed. 'On leaving hospital I had a slight haematoma [clot] on one side, which was painful and I thought I was opening up again because it was red and swollen. It felt like a lump and I've still got a reduced form of it.' (*Jean, two years later*)

'Half an hour before my discharge from hospital [seven days

after the operation] they took the stitches out and the wound went flumf, and opened up. Still trying to be the model patient, I tried to pass it off by saying, "Oh, I'm dripping blood!" I didn't receive any explanation of why it had happened. The nurse just said: "Here are some dressings, off you go!"' (*Jenny*)

She was duly despatched with a wound that was bleeding and leaking 'copious quantities of fluid', and which required a large dressing to be changed by a district nurse, twice daily for five weeks afterwards.

Although it is very unpleasant and very inconvenient, there is no need to worry that when the wound opens in this way, the whole thing is going to burst out! All that happens is that a small area in the wound is slower to heal than the rest, and when the supporting stitches or clips are removed, the wound springs a leak through a hole. This is known as a 'sinus' and will have to be cleaned daily until it gradually disappears as the wound heals over completely.

The three women in our group who had vertical incisions all experienced some problems.

Louise said: 'The bottom two stitches didn't heal; went septic and developed an abcess seven days after my operation. They were going to let me out and they couldn't. They said it would have to burst or they would drain it. They drained it in the end.

'By the time I left it was still very red and sore, but they let me home. I had to go back twice in one week to make sure everything was healing, and for re-dressing. It took a while but it did heal eventually.'

Angela didn't have any problems until two days after she got home, her stitches 'started going septic. They got all red and angry and started to bleed. I thought my stitches were coming undone and everything was going to come out.' [But it didn't.]

Elaine had her stitches out before she left hospital. 'I was sent home with an abcess. They never advised me what to do about it, or how it should be treated. I treated it myself knowing it would get better somehow.' It got better over a couple of months.

Having looked in great detail at the experience of being in hospital, we shall now look at what to expect when you re-enter the outside world.

8

How Long Before I Can Hang Glide?

Leaving hospital

One of the first and often unexpected hurdles after a stay in hospital is making the transition from being a patient to being a person in the outside world again: 'Being in bed in hospital is like being in prison. When you come out you are completely disorientated. Even the pavement comes up to meet you. It's amazing how quickly we lose our understanding of the world.' (*Gynae*)

Simple, everyday tasks can suddenly become alarming as Nikki discovered: 'I stood bewildered on the pavement outside the hospital with no idea how to cross the zebra crossing.'

This disorientation is partly due to the anaesthetic and effects of the operation. It is also a reaction to having been totally dependent on others. Carole described this as the worst moment: 'Leaving the security of the hospital, not knowing what I could and couldn't do.' 'Even for a relatively fit, healthy person, there's a great deal of difficulty in coming to terms with the hospital where you are regimented; you make no decisions about your own welfare; you are fed, clothed, washed and you lose interest in life.' (*Gynae*)

When you re-emerge into the real world, you can feel as if you have been reborn, which will mean you can feel fragile, tearful and vulnerable. You may be able to put a brave face on it, but if you and your family and friends know what to expect, it will be much easier for all of you. It is important that neither you nor those around you expect you to be fully recovered, just because you have left the hospital.

Time to convalesce

'You can be very touchy for the first three days at home. We don't want them to make invalids of themselves, but two weeks' convalescence is very important so we encourage it. It means going away for two weeks. It may not be a very good idea for everyone, depending on the circumstances: some women may not have been away from their family ever before so after being in hospital for twelve days, the thought of another two weeks might make them a little reluctant. They would rather organize things at home.' (*Staff Nurse*)

'As the system is at the moment, there are hundreds of women discharged from hospital after five days, back into traumatic life, with the words "take things easy" without there being any likelihood that they could ever take things easy. Entitlement to assistance is one thing, actually getting it another, and knowing that it might be available another thing again.' (*Jenny*)

Organizing things at home was what most of the interviewees opted for. Home help came in the form of husbands, children, friends, mothers and in one case a paid proxy mother.

'When I came out of hospital, I was allowed to be lazy and my husband did everything for me.' (*Sandra*)

'Luckily, I had my mum and my husband was here as well. I didn't do hardly anything.' (*Carole*)

'Whatever other message my family got, it was that I was to be allowed to do nothing for three months. It was fantastic – all I did was eat my meals and wander around.' (*Angela*)

Louise's mum came to stay for a while and Elaine went to stay with her mother for the summer.

Convalescing at home was especially difficult if there were young children around. For example, Fiona had told her four children that she would be incapacitated for a short while on her return, but as they were only aged between five and ten, they didn't really understand. Her family all expected her to get back to the domestic routine of looking after them all straightaway. The only help she received was from friends.

Jean decided to try and convince her children in another way. 'I stayed in my night clothes for a week after I returned home so that the children realized I was not well.'

Celia chose to come out of hospital earlier because she didn't want her children to be on their own on their half-term holiday. Their planned sitter had let her down so a friend's older children came to the rescue. 'As long as I was up in bed or pottering quietly, they came up and saw me. They were happy and I was perfectly happy. I didn't go up or down stairs for the first three days. It was really very easy.'

Margaret, separated from her husband, stayed with a friend for two weeks immediately after leaving hospital and then went to a new flat. 'I had to return to living alone.'

It is impossible to give a definite programme of recovery as everyone will vary. Six weeks after the operation, Fiona was digging the allotment and Jenny started a new job. Ten weeks afterwards, Sandra was pitching a tent on a camping holiday, although she felt it actually took her six months to fully recover. For Angela it was much longer; she felt it was three years before she was 'able to go through a whole day and an evening without feeling exhausted.'

No one can lay down precise guidelines and say what would be acceptable progress for every woman because everyone responds differently to the trauma. The whole process is much more a matter of trial and error for each woman but there are certain things you can expect to feel at some point during your recovery period. Whatever the individual experience, everyone agrees that you get better in stages.

The first two weeks

For about the first two weeks, you will feel exhausted. Everyone mentioned feeling exceptionally tired at first. This tiredness is often a reaction to going home and picking up where you left off; in your domestic life, your career, coping with bills, making plans for the future. Suddenly you are faced with all sorts of large and small responsibilities which, temporarily, you put out of sight, if not out of mind. This is why it is extremely important to make arrangements *beforehand* for adequate care, not only for yourself but if necessary, for your family.

Because of the practical difficulties that face women when returning home at a time when they are least able to set limits assertively with those around them, some hospitals encourage patients to go to a convalescent home as a way of ensuring two weeks free from worrying about meals or housework.

Jean was offered convalescence but opted for a proxy mother because she wanted to get back to her children. Fiona was also offered the opportunity because she had needed a blood transfusion but she too turned it down because she wanted to get back home.

The only woman we interviewed who had experienced formal convalescence was Sally, who recommended it highly: 'I really think you should go somewhere before going home because when you go home you can't concentrate on what's going on around you. I couldn't plan what to have for tea, I was so wrapped up in what happened to me and worried about the future. You need time for yourself.' Sally's family looked after themselves in her absence. 'I had a friend who came in, did the hoovering . . . generally the children had to do more but I don't think it did them any harm.'

After a disastrous start, Sally raved about the benefits of going away to convalesce. 'Quite a few people wanted to leave as soon as they arrived. It was like a women's prison. They didn't have any messing about with anybody. I climbed forty-five stairs three days after I left the hospital: younger women on the top floor, older women below. We made a pact: we'll give it three days and if it's awful, we'll go home.

'We went to our first meal. Those that had been there longer came up and said, "When the going gets tough, don't give up. Don't let them beat you. It's really worth it once you get through it all. You'll be glad you stayed." We couldn't see this at all at the time. We thought we were being punished. We got on the phone to home crying. Anyway, we got through the first three days and then we said, we'll give it a week. We stayed for two weeks! We went out for walks every day, building up gradually, ten, fifteen, twenty minutes. In the end we were going for hour-long walks.

It was up and down hill; you went off with someone who was ahead of you, and you wanted to keep up with them so you increased. By the second week, we were a lot more mobile and mentally better. The following week, another influx of patients arrived and we told them what we had been told and there they were on the phone, like we had been! After the two weeks, I came home and was raring to go. I really felt well – as though I had been on holiday.'

Whether or not you are offered convalescence seems to depend not only on your hospital but on the surgeon in charge of you. The Staff Nurse reported that in her hospital, one consultant who had had a hysterectomy herself didn't think it necessary to convalesce so didn't encourage it, whereas another consultant included the medical social worker on his ward round to ensure all his patients were offered the opportunity.

The Staff Nurse thought it especially important for older women to get away and also those women she knew were returning to a chaotic household with young children. Many of her patients enjoyed their two weeks away: 'They are not holiday camps but they are nice, well organized places by the sea. They can go for long walks and there's someone to look after them. One place is run by monks and the postcards we get from past patients are quite hilarious.'

If you want to enquire about possibilities yourself, you could follow up some of Sandra's recommendations. As a health visitor, she too recommended a period away and told us that there are many homes belonging to charities, unions and the Civil Service for employees and their relatives. She suggested that the occupational health nurse at work or the medical social worker at the hospital would have this information.

The first two months

A landmark in the first two months after the operation is the six-week check-up with the gynaecologist. Whereas you may be treading cautiously beforehand, the gynaecologist's 'all clear' may give you a sharp burst of renewed confidence and make you more adventurous.

This meeting should give you the opportunity to check on your progress and clear up any queries you may have about your recovery.

Bleeding

One of the first symptoms which worries many women during the first few weeks or months after leaving hospital is vaginal bleeding. If you are not warned that this might happen, you might panic and think everything is falling out! It is quite normal to have a slight bloodstained or yellow discharge soon after the operation. Usually, this discharge stops within three weeks but sometimes it may go on longer and could be an indication of something more serious. The discharge can be caused by a little pocket of fluid and debris which collects at the top of the vagina and then bursts; sometimes the bleeding comes from the line of stitches at the top of your vagina; or else it can occur because you get little bubbles of tissues like warts which form as the skin heals inside and these can bleed and discharge. No one knows how to prevent them and they can last for a few months and can be cauterized. You may find that a discharge is intermittent and occurs for a couple of days over a period of several months.

'I bled for ten weeks after the operation. It was a yellow discharge and I had to wear a pad every day. I went to the doctor because I was worried and she said it was just all the muck coming out.' (*Carole*)

'I bled for a while after coming home. I went to the doctor because I thought I had an infection but it turned sort of yellowy, not blood any more. When I brought it up at my next six-week check-up with the gynaecologist, he told me, "Wear pads if it's that bad." I got the impression he didn't think it worth talking about . . . It was quite a long time because I remember trying out all the different kinds of pads.' (*Margaret*)

If the bleeding becomes heavy, or the discharge has a smell, or even if you are just worried, it would be wise to check it out with your GP.

Tiredness

Whether you have been convalescing at home or away you will probably find that the tiredness continues, not all the time but in patches. Many women expressed feeling suddenly overwhelmed and exhausted: sometimes they were surprised and impatient with themselves.

'I used to get furious because I felt so tired. I don't like being ill. I used to cry with frustration at not being able to do things.' (*Fiona*)

'The tiredness amazed me. I couldn't believe how long it took to want to get up and do anything. When my friend went to work, she'd say, "Make yourself a coffee". She'd come in at lunchtime and I'd still be sitting there waiting for my coffee. I hadn't moved!' (*Margaret*)

'I found it very difficult to sit there and do nothing. I'm a houseproud person and felt I wanted to get on and do something but I felt completely drained. No physical strength of any kind.' (*Louise*)

'Take it very gently and carefully and do what you feel you can do and no more. If you feel you can peel half the potatoes, don't think, "Well, I can finish them," go and sit. Your body will tell you what you can take and what you can't.' (*Celia*)

'I couldn't write properly. I've got big writing anyway but it was just ginormous! I didn't feel as though I had any control over the pen. I had difficulty writing for about five weeks afterwards. It was a hassle to concentrate. I love reading normally but I used to get terribly tired and couldn't remember what I had read.' (*Fiona*)

Pacing your activity during the day is very important. 'By mid-afternoon, I was tired so I used to have a sleep – otherwise it was hopeless.' (*Louise*)

'When you've lived below par for so long you get used to it. And suddenly you find you have a lot of energy; you use it too quickly and woomph, you go down again.' (*Sandra*)

'I used to feel fine in the morning, and then about eleven o'clock, I used to feel jagged around the edges. I worked out a system. All the kids were at school so I put my feet up from eleven till one, then I felt better. I may not have slept but I read and sometimes slept. Then I could keep going until about five. Then I'd had it and would have to sit down for most of the evening.' (*Fiona*)

Even up to several weeks after the operation, you can still be subject to unaccountable and unexpected periods of exhaustion. Although some of the women were warned that they would feel tired, they couldn't believe the extent of it. Even though the spirit may have been willing, the flesh was often still too weak!

'Recovery is not quick but women expect it to be quick, it's what they hope.' (*Gynae*) For this reason, women find themselves pushing a little too hard, too soon. Two weeks after the operation Jean went to a wedding reception opposite. 'I felt incredibly shaky when I put proper clothes on. There was rush matting on the floor and I thought, "God, I mustn't fall over." I had one slow dance with M and came straight home. I did it because I needed to prove to myself that I could.' Jean learned her lesson from not proceeding more cautiously: 'It caught up with me about six months afterwards. I was exhausted, shaky, numb. Don't run before you can walk.'

There is a fine balance between pushing yourself too quickly and doing yourself harm in the long run, and on the other hand treating yourself too much like an invalid and not making any effort at all. The solution is to see recovery as a *very gradual process*.

This is why it is preferable to use other people's advice as a guide rather than feeling you have to meet a deadline: 'I had been *told* I would feel a different women in six months. I didn't get out of the house for four months by which time, according to the theorists, I should have been back at school, doing the Highland Fling! But that was very far from the truth.' (*Angela*) 'Do whatever you feel you are up to doing that doesn't give you any discomfort, but nevertheless, push yourself onwards.' (*Gynae*)

The best guide of all is your own body. If you listen to its inner wisdom you'll know what you can and cannot do; you'll know that if you start something too ambitious, you can give yourself permission to stop. Even under normal circumstances, women find it extremely difficult to admit to being tired, as if this in some way shows them to be less than perfect. But trying to be superwoman too early can be disastrous: it's better to go little by little.

'During that time, I would get up and peel a potato, then collapse in a heap and leave the rest. I'd have to do a little bit and sit; do a little bit and sit. As the days went by, I found I was doing two things and then sitting and then three things and then sitting and so on.' Four weeks after her operation Celia thought she could cope with the shopping but found it 'absolute hell. I was so tired at the end of it, walking around the supermarket, loading the car. I went out on my own as I thought I'd feel all right but it was coming home that I didn't feel as good as I had thought. I came home in a soggy heap.' This happened a couple of times before she could really cope with it.

Five weeks afterwards Ellen had a similar experience. 'I went down to the village because I felt I had got this energy and wanted to go to the bank. I knew when I got there that I was really tired. I started back, got to a seat, collapsed on it and just couldn't get myself home. I felt really frustrated and weepy. A friend stopped and said, "Gosh, you look awful!", and gave me lift home. I was pushing myself too much but at the time I felt I wanted to do it.'

Even short, familiar walks can be too much. The first time Fiona went out on her own was to the corner shop for some cigarettes: 'I went down the back garden path and felt perfectly all right. I opened the back gate and suddenly I couldn't move. I couldn't go out. I turned round and came back thinking "You stupid fool, what on earth's the matter with you?" I tried again, four times I tried but couldn't get beyond the back gate. I felt all hot and weak and everything drained away. So I went back and sat down and thought, "Why don't you want to go?" I think it was because I was on my own, I'd been out before but always with someone, so I thought I would take the dog. I put him on a lead and I hoped he wouldn't pull me over. I went out of the back gate and went down to the shop. I was perfectly all right. It never happened again.'

Whatever you attempt at this time, it is important to remember that you will be incapable of doing some of the things that you normally do and that however much you are warned of this, you will still be taken by surprise. Louise, for example, had been told to expect activities like washing and shopping to be tiring but she didn't anticipate at times not being able 'to lift a duster'.

In the second month, your body will be able to cope with a variety of activities ranging from cooking, ironing and vacuuming to swimming, horse-riding and motorcycling. Any activity which *gently* strenghtens your abdominal muscles is recommended. Some women are given a series of exercises to follow while they are in hospital to tone up these muscles. Nikki learned during the course of the interviews that her present 'tummy' could have been avoided in this way and since this is one of the longer-lasting side effects of abdominal surgery, we recommend that you ask the hospital physiotherapist to give you some appropriate exercises.

Lifting

Most women are cautioned against lifting anything more than a kettle full of water for the first month and heavier objects for at least *three* months after surgery. This is to give the *internal* healing time to occur. 'I think most women think it's healed on the outside and they just don't realize how much needlework and stitchery has gone on, on the inside.' (*Sandra*)

Sally used the scar colour as a guide: 'Unless you have something to look at, you don't know how well healed you are. When your scar is white (or darker depending on your skin pigment), you are completely healed inside. All the time it's pink, there are still some healing processes going on.' Margaret remembered 'pin-prick sensations' in her scar for months afterwards which can be expected as the tissue heals together inside.

The inside stitches take about six weeks to dissolve. If you strain this part of your body, your abdomen becomes sore and uncomfortable. In order to avoid over-straining, certain activities must be approached with great care: be careful of lifting or taking a young child in your arms or onto your lap. If the child falls, you will instinctively move to save them and, in doing so, may damage yourself. It is better to sit the child beside you. Similarly, if you do go swimming, use the steps – never jump or dive into the water.

Lifting and stretching can all strain the delicate internal needlework which is why even bedmaking should be avoided for the same reason. If it is necessary to lift something, place your feet apart, bend your knees, keeping your back straight, hold the object to be lifted or carried close to your body and lift by straightening your knees rather than pulling upwards with your arms.

Driving

Don't drive too soon. If you have to brake suddenly, your internal stitches may overstretch or snap. It is usually considered safe to drive four to six weeks after surgery, but it is important to remember the following:

- Getting in and out of the car needs to be done carefully, especially a small or low car.
- Coping with traffic may become one of the normal tasks which can suddenly overwhelm you. You need to wait until you have enough confidence to tackle it, but don't wait so long that you lose confidence altogether!
- Your concentration may also be impaired, so long car journeys require a stop every hour. This applies even if you are the passenger on a long car ride: you must avoid sitting too long in one position because your abdominal muscles can stiffen up and become uncomfortable. Stretch yourself regularly.

Back to work

'Women who say to me: "I'm going back to work after six or eight weeks," I just tell them they're fools. However well you feel at eight weeks, and even though employers expect women to do it, I think it's wrong to go back to a full-time job so soon.' Sandra felt that it took twelve weeks to get back together again.

Obviously, the right time to return to work will depend on the individual and the work involved. Even though Jenny had started a new job six weeks after her operation, she admitted that it would have been better to wait a bit longer. The severe anaemia Angela was suffering from at the time of her surgery meant a much longer recovery period. She had six months off from her teaching job but even after that she said, 'It really knocked the stuffing out of me.'

Louise started slowly: 'I went part-time for a couple of hours a day through an agency and eventually I got back on my feet.' Margaret, too, started by working half a day until she felt able to go back full-time.

The first year

In reply to the question "How long do you think it takes to recover fully from the operation?', we received the following answers:

'The gynaecologist said it would take three months to recover but it actually took six to get better.' (*Celia*)

'It was six to nine months before I felt better. It was close on a year before I felt fit enough to play badminton. The tiredness continued for months and months.' (*Margaret*)

'I was told it would take a year to get over it totally and it did.' (*Jean*)

'It took six months to get back into things.' (*Elaine*)

'Frankly, it's taken me almost a year to say, "Yes, I feel like my old self." It could be longer before you reap the benefit, you have to be patient.' (*Sally*)

'After six months, I had more energy than I ever had before and I kept going up and up.' (*Ellen*)

'I have certainly emotionally and physically recovered. It probably took about a year.' (*Jenny*)

From their answers it appears that, although it may be sooner and although recovery will depend on all sorts of factors, the first year should see you fully recovered and able to put your hysterectomy firmly behind you!

9
The Aftermath

The following are commonly thought to be possible long-term after-effects of hysterectomy. We look at these in the light of the women's actual experience.

Weight gain

Elaine experienced 'slight' weight gain. Sandra gained weight and Carole, too, put on weight. She described herself as having no willpower to diet. 'It's only because we're going on holiday in August that I'm trying to do something about it now.'

On the other hand, Louise lost 24 pounds (11 kilos). Fiona, too, lost weight: 'I never put it back on. I'd always had a "pot" and that went completely. I used to do the old exercises we did in hospital: lying on the bed, raising your legs up in the air and letting them down again slowly. Roll round and round in the bed over one side, and back to the other. That tones up all the muscles. They said to continue with that when you got home, so I did.'

Constipation, loss of appetite and wind

Angela thought she no longer has the capacity to eat the way she did before: 'I don't think my alimentary canal has ever recovered [after four years]. Wind is a problem I've retained. If they were to ask me now, "Have you passed wind?", I'd say "Yes, and I haven't stopped since!"' Jean said that eating meat gave her a lot of wind, but she had put that down to getting older [she was 33!].

'I've been left a permanent legacy of digestive problems and intermittent wind, which I never had in my life before.' (*Nikki*)

Somewhat luckier was Margaret, for whom the situation was reversed. 'Since the operation I've definitely noticed that I have not suffered any constipation, and I was very prone to it before.'

It is very understandable after your innards have been rearranged during the operation, that your bowels/intestines will reflect this rearrangement in a changed pattern of digestion.

Headaches

Carole reported headaches only *since* the operation, and Margaret, too, had 'headaches, and I didn't have them before the operation. I used to have them every day, I lived on Anadin, but they've stopped over the last few months.'

Conversely, Celia said that she suffered a lot of headaches before the operation but *stopped* having them afterwards. So did Angela: 'The one thing it did for me was get rid of my headaches. I had a permanent headache before, and I haven't had one since.'

Disturbed sleep and tiredness

Sandra suffered from disturbed sleep, as did Celia, for eighteen months following the operation. Two years afterwards, Carole described the problem as 'terrible. Ever since the operation I wake up every night; sometimes staying awake for hours on end. I'm a really bad sleeper now, whereas I was really good before.' This contributes to her current continual tiredness. 'I got really tired after my operation. Even now [two years later] if I sit down in the warm of an evening, I'll nod off for twenty minutes.'

Celia's experience was similar: 'Tiredness now [three years later] quite a bit of the time. I'm much more conscious of being tired now. I fall asleep in front of the telly when I never used to.'

Hair growth

Extra hair growth is another popular belief after hysterectomy. Only two of our group mentioned this – Ellen and Elaine grew more facial hair, but for both of them it coincided with the menopause rather than as a result of hysterectomy.

Absentmindedness – memory loss

After her own experience of memory lapse, which has since become a pattern, Nikki was concerned to know whether anyone else had suffered similar lapses in memory.

Celia recognized the symptom but had put it down to age, and Jean recognized it, not after hysterectomy but as something that happened after the birth of each of her three children. This possibly links the condition to hormonal changes in our metabolism.

It's difficult to make a direct connection between hysterectomy and memory loss, although it is very likely that a change in hormonal levels could contribute to headaches, weight loss and disturbed sleep.

Nabothian follicle

This is one final possible after-effect. If the cervix is retained, a normal occurrence is the growth of a follicle or cyst which acts like a harmless blister – an ingenious way of protecting the wound from infection. The cervix produces a mucus which acts as a defensive barrier against bacteria. Sometimes the mucus, being thick and sticky, blocks the mouth of the cervix, causing it to swell up.

It is quite painless, but its appearance can be misleading if you or your GP think it is indicative of something much worse. Eventually, the Nabothian follicle goes 'pop' and out comes the mucus through the vagina.

Looking at the after-effects of hysterectomy, it is necessary to take into account other factors which complicate the issue. Although connections may be assumed between certain symptoms and the operation, it is difficult to predict accurately what will happen over the longer term. The after-effects of hysterectomy on a woman's own perception of her recovery will depend on a diversity of factors, including her treatment in hospital at the hands of the surgeon and other medical staff; whether the symptom for which she originally had the hysterectomy has since recurred; her attitude to having a hysterectomy in the first place; and whether or not she needs to rely on prolonged medication after surgery.

In this sense, every woman's experience is unique. But before we look at how you can help yourself towards rapid recovery, we will describe the circumstances of five women which have had a marked effect on their sense of overall recovery from the operation. We felt it important to include them, not because they give an indication of what could generally be expected after hysterectomy, but because what happened to them could easily happen to anyone in similar circumstances.

Rough handling in theatre

'I have been left with a permanent back problem right at the base of my spine – somewhere around my coccyx [tail bone]. I could hardly walk.' Apart from crippling pain, Angela was even more annoyed that, when she asked for help, no one would accept responsibility for the problem.

'The gynae people just didn't want to know, and denied it was anything to do with the operation. But talking to a gynaecologist friend of ours later, he said, "it's not uncommon. It's the way people are banged on to the trolleys."' Angela went to various people for help, was put on anti-inflammatory drugs to stop the pain. She was told she would recover in time, but it was a major disability for a year after her operation. 'It's certainly a lot better now, but it's a permanent legacy. I didn't want to take drugs for ever so I now have a hot water bottle when it gets really bad, and gear my life accordingly.'

Recurrence of former symptom

'A year later the PID [pelvic inflammatory disease, see pages 32-3] process appeared to become reactivated, I had pain again, considerable abdominal distension and more adhesions.' Jenny had woken from her operation to find that the surgeon had not removed all of her womb but had left a section of her uterus intact. His personal values were very strong. 'He felt that for any woman of a child-bearing age to be in a position where physically she was unable to conceive was an absolute disaster.' Because of this attitude he left Jenny physically able to conceive (for an egg to become attached to the remaining section of uterine wall), but of course, spontaneous abortion followed straightaway. Likewise, she continued to menstruate. Each month she faced the possibility of getting pregnant and then immediately aborting.

The strength of the surgeon's personal values seems to have outweighed the consideration for the physical and psychological welfare of his patient. Understandably, she sought the help of another gynaecologist. 'The turning point came when I saw the second gynaecologist and I felt I had reclaimed the situation. That made a tremendous difference to the speed of recovery.' She later underwent another operation to clip her Fallopian tubes so as to prevent any possibility at all of conception and stop her worrying every month.

The acute pain in Carole's right side flared up again eighteen months after her hysterectomy. She was sent for a further body scan because it was thought there may be trouble with an ovary. But: 'On the scan they couldn't find the left ovary at all. The doctor couldn't understand why it wasn't visible. The right ovary was a bit swollen, but when Mr W examined me he said everything was normal. They say that there's nothing wrong whatsoever.'

Carole went on: 'What I have in the back of my mind is, I had this pain before my hysterectomy and I still have it. It's their way of saying, "Well that's it. We've not made a mistake. OK, you've still got the pain but forget about it." Really and truly, all it's done is stop the heavy periods.' So Carole's pain persists, with no one being able to offer a medical explanation. 'The pain doesn't happen at any particular time. I could just be sitting there and all of a sudden it goes '*zhunk*' and it's there. It really aches, you can't forget it. One day I got stuck in my chair. I keep saying to my husband, "They say there's nothing wrong. But how can it be in my mind when it's so painful?"'

It is impossible to say if and how Carole's undoubted physical pain is affected by anything else in her life. Whatever the reason, she is still in pain, and no one knows why.

Ambivalence to hysterectomy

Louise found it very hard to adjust to the fact that she could no longer have children. Since the birth of her daughter, eight years before, she had been trying unsuccessfully to get pregnant, but each time she had miscarried. Louise had to make her mind up on the spot, in very unsupportive circumstances. In her own words, 'It all happened very quickly. I plumped for hysterectomy which I wished I hadn't. But I did. I was still desperately trying for another child and I knew if I had a hysterectomy it was finished, there would be no going back. Four days later I was in there.'

The lack of time to make a clear decision must have contributed to the unhappiness she felt after the operation. 'I bottled most of it up inside. I was tearful and depressed for months. My mum stayed for a while, but after a few weeks I wanted to be on my own. There was something I had to sort out for myself. She couldn't begin to sense how I felt because she had not had a hysterectomy. In the end, my mum reluctantly went home. I sorted myself out. Not very well, but I managed. I still had an eight-year-old daughter to look after, regardless. The doctor at the hospital told me to take a part-time job as a start. He said if I didn't, I probably would have a breakdown. I did what he said and eventually I got back on my feet.'

Louise's legacy is still not being able to come to terms with not having another child. 'I would be a liar if I said I didn't want more children even now. I do, I would dearly love one. I asked my sister to have one for me, but she refused.'

Continuing medication

Sally had both ovaries removed and, with her natural hormone supply gone, she was dependent on an artificial source. This is called HRT (Hormone Replacement Therapy), which we'll look at more fully in Chapter 11 where we consider all the implications of HRT.

Sally's situation provides one example of what can happen. Having hormone problems is often dismissed: 'Doctors still say it's only a hormone imbalance. But to say that is ridiculous, because it affects your whole life. Everything about you. It's as crucial as your blood supply.'

After four years of ovarian pain and considerable discomfort and the removal of one ovary without subsequent improvement, Sally was offered hysterectomy as a last resort.

Probably because hormone therapy is at an experimental stage, neither she nor her doctor could anticipate the emotional ups and downs corresponding to hormonal changes.

'They don't tell you about the depression. I got very weepy and lost a lot of weight. I got very gaunt in the face and I couldn't look in the mirror. I couldn't bear to look at myself. I really thought I had changed. I kept finding fault all the time.'

A lot of Sally's practical difficulties obtaining medication, the side effects of using HRT, the attitude of the medical profession who prescribe it, are all discussed later on in detail. The uncertainty about HRT fuels her own uncertainty about her future and prevents her feeling a full sense of recovery. 'When I get my hormone problem sorted out completely, I know I shall be all right. But at the moment, it's so up and down, it's stopping me really benefitting.'

10

Sex and Sexuality

Sex, as the Staff Nurse said, is 'the priority question' – one which is often on a patient's mind even if she finds it difficult to ask. Some women are concerned about their sexual response:

- Is my sex drive going to be changed by the removal of my womb?

Some women are worried about the effect of surgery on their genitals:

- What will I be like inside?
- Will my vagina feel any different to my husband during intercourse?

Others are concerned to know when they will be able to make love again:

- When will it be safe to have sex again after surgery?
- Is there any danger of doing any damage?

Sexual drive and response

Sexual drive is the need or wish for sexual contact and sexual response is our ability to enjoy that contact. Obviously, one goes with the other – we're not likely to want more of an experience which we don't enjoy and leaves us cold. In looking at how hysterectomy affects sexual activity, a woman's attitude to sex before her operation will have to be taken into consideration. If, in the past, a woman has found that sex generally wasn't much fun anyway, or just something she felt she had to put up with, then she could well find the same after hysterectomy as before.

Although none of our interviewees reported a long-term lack of interest in sex before the operation, several mentioned that the pleasure had gone out of sex in the recent past because of all the symptoms they were suffering. Intercourse had often been difficult and they had withdrawn from sexual contact because of the pain.

'We couldn't make love at all because it was so painful. I knew that when we made love it would be hell so we tended not to because C wasn't getting any satisfaction and I certainly wasn't.' (*Celia*)

'Before [hysterectomy] it was excruciatingly painful as my womb was so distended. When we made love I used to wish the bed had a dip in it. I didn't feel clean, I was in pain. It killed any sort of sexual pleasure and therefore if I turned over on my side of the bed, and he turned over on his side of the bed and gave me a cuddle, I thought, "Oh my God, he's going to ask me to make love," which is awful. We went on like that for nearly a year. I was incredibly distant from M but I didn't want to be.' Not surprisingly, Jean's sex life became virtually non-existent.

'The pain came from penetration because it was banging up against the cervix. I kept pulling away; I used to be going up the bed as he was going into me.' (*Fiona*)

'I had always had problems with penetration because of my cervix. I had this inflamed cervix and no one had seen it when they examined me. I could have had it for more than five years. I had trouble with sexual intercourse for a long time. In certain positions it was excruciatingly painful.' (*Sally*)

'I had considerable pain on orgasm as a result of the adhesions. I was also bleeding fairly constantly and in a lot of pain.' (*Jenny*) Alleviation of this pain was a prime factor in Jenny seeking help.

Sexual response

In order to understand fully how hysterectomy can affect our sexual response, we must understand the basics of normal sexual arousal.

All sorts of triggers can start the process of sexual arousal. As we become aroused various changes occur in our bodies, especially in the pelvic area. Extra blood starts flowing which cause our genitals to swell and our vaginas to lubricate.

Before arousal the vagina is 3½-4 inches (8-10cm) long, and the vaginal walls lie together touching each other, like two sheets on a bed. It is only when something enters the vagina, such as a penis in intercourse, or a speculum in an internal examination, or when something leaves the vagina like a baby, that the walls part and fold themselves around the object, just like sheets fold around someone lying in the bed. The vaginal walls are very elastic and can stretch very wide.

Another of the effects of sexual arousal, although we are not always aware of it, is the lengthening of the vagina. It balloons out so that instead of being its usual length, it is temporarily increased to 5 or 6 inches (13-15cm).

Orgasm

If you are aroused enough, and there is enough tension in your pelvis caused by all that extra blood, then you may experience orgasm, which is a release of this tension. The contractions in orgasm occur in the uterus and the vagina, but unless you are heavily pregnant, you are unlikely to feel them in the uterus. The contractions that most of us recognize are those of the vaginal muscle which stretches along the crotch from the pubic bone at the top, to the coccyx or tail bone at the bottom. (This is called the pubococcygeal, or pc muscle for short.) This muscle includes your clitoris at the top of the vagina, and the vaginal opening itself. When it comes to sensitivity to pleasure, you will find that the outer part of your vagina, the first third in fact, is highly sensitive to touch of any kind. The inner part of your vagina has no nerve endings, so you cannot feel anything deep inside.

Although there are no touch sensitive nerve endings inside the vagina, it is possible to feel pressure particularly against the cervix.

One of the awful vicious circles about lack of sexual pleasure is the less aroused you are, the less aroused you can be. If you agree to make love when you don't want to and when it hurts, then your body will not begin to get sexually aroused, and any potential pleasure will be spoiled by painful sensations. This is why if you are not aroused, and the vagina doesn't expand, the pressure on the cervix will be painful in some positions.

After hysterectomy

If you have an abdominal hysterectomy and if your cervix is removed, your vagina will have a little seam of stitches right at the top. If you retain your cervix, your vagina will be completely unchanged inside. If you have had part of your vagina removed, then the vagina will be shortened a little in length and will also have a seam at the top.

When women are worried about enjoyment of intercourse after hysterectomy, they are usually concerned about their ability to feel anything, their ability to have an orgasm, and the difference it will make to their partners' enjoyment.

With your clitoris and your vagina intact, your sexual response will remain the same. Your capacity to experience orgasm need not be affected at all because your clitoris is untouched and even though the uterus is gone, as you probably didn't feel the contractions before, it isn't going to make much difference. The vaginal contractions are unaffected.

Finally, as your vagina will continue to expand if you are sexually aroused, a man is not going to be able to feel any difference inside, because it is very distended and it is unusual in normal circumstances for a man to feel the cervix during intercourse. If the cervix is removed, as he didn't feel it in the first place, he is not going to notice the change physically. The sensations that a man receives on his penis are much more to do with the entrance of the vagina and this is totally unaffected by hysterectomy.

So, given the facts, there isn't much reason why sex should be less pleasurable than before. But getting aroused and enjoying yourself sexually faces the major obstacle of anxiety. Any kind of anxiety makes it extremely difficult to relax and inhibits our bodies' normal responses to pleasure. For this reason it is very important to talk, to ask questions, not only of the medical staff but also discuss it with your partner. It is a time when everyone needs a lot of reassurance.

Not all the women we interviewed felt able to ask for such information. 'In hospital we all wanted to ask when it would be all right, but no one could pluck up the courage. No one had been told.' (*Sally*) She eventually asked the sister who told them: '"Not normally until you've had your post-op check-up." Since then we've all been told different things and read different things.'

After a lot of hesitation, Jean approached her doctor because of her anxiety. 'I was terribly worried that when we made love, the seam at the top would burst and M would go through! The doctor's reply to that was "put it like this, unless you've got an exceptionally well-endowed husband, or a complete freak, you're all right.'' I was able to laugh about it afterwards with M.'

Ellen turned to a friend for some answers: 'I was trying to find out what sex would be like afterwards but it was difficult to obtain such personal information. What information I did get from my friend, I treasured, as I knew it had been very hard for her to talk about.'

A wider perspective

Although there is no physical reason why you should feel less like sex following surgery, deep down we know that sex isn't just a question of technicalities. Up until now, we have focused on the mechanics of sexual activity.

However, our interest in and enjoyment of sex and sexual activity are also dependent on how we feel about our bodies, our feelings towards our partners, on whether or not we are relaxed, whether we are with a partner who is putting pressure on or being patient, and on our mental and physical health. All these factors make the concerns about sex after hysterectomy more complex but much more realistic.

Given our dependence on approval from others, a woman after hysterectomy may be concerned that her male partner might find her less attractive and therefore less sexually desirable. There is a myth that some men believe 'it's not much fun having sex with a woman who has had a hysterectomy. It's not supposed to be as exciting. The excitement comes from the fact that there is a possibility the woman might conceive.' (*Gynae*)

Our image of ourselves can easily be swayed by how someone else sees us. Since our self-image is so closely bound up with our social image – how we look, how feminine we are – having a scar and no longer having a womb can often make many women feel unattractive and redundant. There is no reason why you should feel like this, especially if you are proud of your body and of the person you are. This is influenced as well by your partner's attitude towards you and women in general.

'The involvement of the man depends very much on his psyche; on his understanding of female genitals; on their relationship, whether it is one of love, adoration, affection, respect. Or whether they have sex out of pique, envy, greed. It is so profound. And the woman's responses and recovery will really depend on the man to a great extent.' (*Gynae*)

Jean described some men as being 'womb men'. She summed up the situation by saying that '. . . there are legs men, tits men, and womb men. If you've got a womb man, you'll be in a lot of trouble!'

None of the women we interviewed reported their partners to be less sexually attracted to them as a result of hysterectomy.

'E didn't view me any differently, I didn't talk about it with him because he's not that interested. As long as you're upright and not visibly deformed in any way, that's as far as he goes.' (*Fiona*)

'My husband was very supportive anyway, so he wasn't funny about it, as I gather some men are.' (*Celia*)

'He was worried about whether I would be able to cope with feeling pathetic and weak, or overdoing it. He was worried about that but not about my losing my femininity.' (*Jean*)

It is difficult to identify exactly what it is that makes a woman feel a woman and feminine. It must vary with each individual. It could be rooted in an attractive image, an ability to bear children, the capacity to 'turn on' her partner or something more deeply rooted in her own sense of self.

Louise described herself as a 'freak' afterwards because she couldn't have any more children and was very unhappy about that. Sally said she felt less of a woman when at first she found herself unable to respond sexually in the way she had done before. But these feelings were not due to their partners finding them less attractive.

Taking the plunge

Understandably, the main hurdle was the first time! Some women had been told to wait eleven weeks, some eight, others six and others to wait until after their check-up. But not everyone waited. Although Sally had been told to wait for eleven weeks, she was curious so, about six weeks after, she decided to take the plunge and stop 'putting off the evil day'. She thought it was similar to experiencing sex after childbirth: 'It's just like when you've had a baby. You are unsure of how you are going to feel.'

Fiona also took the initiative because she found the anticipation 'a bit daunting. I thought I had better make a move, otherwise I'll never get round to it.' She wasn't so much worried about internal damage but more about the possibility of an over-enthusiastic surgeon: 'I wasn't frightened about bursting open. I was much more frightened that he'd sewn me up and that E wouldn't be able to get in. I thought, if he's stitched me up too tight, what will happen then? But it was all right!'

Sometimes the waiting period before sexual intercourse crystallizes the difference in sexual needs between men and women. Slightly tongue in cheek, the gynaecologist commented: 'You know what men are like, they want to do it anywhere, all the time and as often as they can. And as soon as they've done it, it's over! A woman's sexual responses are different, she wants more from it than a man, much more from it than a man.'

More seriously, it is still easy to fall into the trap of believing that sex isn't sex without a fuck: 'A lot more counselling needs to be done with husbands and boyfriends. They need to know that they must be more gentle when penetrating. It may be dry. It may take time before you get used to having sex again. A lot of them don't realize that you can make love without having intercourse, they don't think of options. And if you mention things like oral sex, they think it's awful. Some men just want vaginal sex, and if they can't have that, it's too bad.' (*Sandra*)

At times like this when two people's needs are different, it is important to *talk* to each other, and avoid anything you are not quite ready for.

'In terms of going back to being sexual, it was almost inadvertent. After about three weeks J was climbing the walls with lust and it was a sort of mercy fuck the first couple of times. And then it actually began to feel okay.' (*Jenny*)

At the time Jenny felt protective of herself, 'enclosed and finding it difficult to give out at all. I was very sensitive to being touched, which I put down to the fact I was leaking, messy, feeling foul about myself. I was very protective of my belly. For quite a long time afterwards I slept with a pillow in front of my tummy, which was physically necessary for about a month, and emotionally necessary for very much longer.'

The need to take time, to use an extra lubricant (like KY jelly) if necessary, the need for sensitivity, care and lack of pressure are paramount at this time. This is particularly so for the first few experiences of intercourse. However reassuring her partner might be, a woman will inevitably feel anxious about what may happen. Anxiety is the biggest passion killer of all, so communication is essential, each step of the way. Her partner may also feel anxious and both people can be disconcerted if, after the first time, there is a little blood or a bit of stitch or a slight discharge. This need not be alarming and is best handled with humour and practical care.

You can consider sexual options other than intercourse as a way of giving pleasure to one another, and if you have had an abdominal hysterectomy, it is also sensible to use a position which avoids discomfort when you make love, by using any way other than on top, for example, lying side by side. And even if you have been told that you won't feel any different inside, you will still probably want to know that first hand. You could always feel with your finger inside your vagina yourself, or look inside with a speculum. But given that most women are reluctant to do either of these things, it could be important to check it out with your partner.

Louise didn't and so was never quite sure: 'I still felt I had this hole. Every time we made love, I said to my boyfriend, "where's the hole?" But he never said how he found it inside, whether it was any different. I never found out. To this day I don't know.'

Jean asked: 'I was terrified he'd notice a difference but M says I don't feel any different and he wouldn't lie to me. He said if anything, it was better because I was tighter inside.'

Minuses and pluses

Apart from the immediate effects, we also asked women whether they felt a hysterectomy had had any long term consequences for their sexual enjoyment.

A year after her operation, Sally was beginning to return to the way she was, after her initial disappointment at her lack of response. 'I tried to hide it from my husband that I felt disappointed. It frightened me because I felt, if I feel like this now, will I always feel this way? I couldn't really ask anyone. I ended up discussing it with women in my self-help group. They brought it up at the hospital when I went for my implant. They said, "how's your love life?" I said, "all right I suppose." They said, "that's not what we hear from most patients: they say it's terrible when they have an implant." I was so surprised. I said, "I must admit, I don't have the same urges that I used to have." That was when I was on the oestrogen-only dosage and they offered to give me testosterone to increase my libido. I must admit it did improve but it still wasn't as it should be. It took me a good six months afterwards before I began to feel like I used to. And it's only a month since orgasm's been good again. I wasn't prepared for that.'

Sally's experience underlines the importance of communication rather than struggling through it alone. She continued: 'I know one woman whose husband has left her because she had similar problems sexually. I think he felt that because she wasn't interested in him, that was part of the 'package'. They didn't have the kind of relationship where you talk about things like that.

'I didn't open up at the beginning to my husband, I kept quiet but I supposed he must have sensed something. He never made any demands on me. He never said, "What's the matter with you?", or "Snap out of it!" Nothing like that. I never made the first moves. I would rather watch a good film on television and stayed up as late as I could, any excuse. You can't let it go on like that and lots of women do.'

Obviously, Sally's hormone treatment is a contributing factor to her own experience. There is no way of predicting how a hysterectomy will affect a woman's sexual feelings. Especially when our sexual responses are so easily influenced by other emotions and concerns in our lives.

Louise remarked on the difference in the women who had been in hospital with her: 'We all seemed to have different reactions. One couldn't get enough of it, the other one accepted it for what it was, but I was totally and utterly switched off.' She said that it was eighteen months before she felt like sex again. 'It hurt for a long time, unless it was in my mind. It was very, very painful and I wanted to get it over and done with quickly. If I'm honest, I'm still dubious about sex. But I don't know if it's to do with hysterectomy or the fact that I wanted another child and I never had it. I never fulfilled that one thing. And I'm not going to fulfil it now. My attitude is, you have sex to have children. If you can't have children, why bother to have sex?'

Margaret was separated from her husband at the time of her operation, so she didn't have any sexual contact for a long time: 'Then we started getting back together again and it was painful. It took a year before it wasn't so painful. Even now, there's the odd time when I can feel pain on intercourse, not so intense but the same, whatever causes it.' She added, 'I think I lost the inclination to have sex. I don't attribute that to hysterectomy, just to getting old!'

At the time of her interview, Carole was still suffering from a sexual difficulty. 'Everything was okay after the operation, it was okay for a year but slowly it got worse and worse, until there's nothing there. Nothing at all. I can't feel anything. I can't understand what's happening because it didn't happen straightaway. My GP said, "Sometimes when you have big operations it does happen. It upsets your hormones." I would have expected that immediately afterwards, not two years later. She referred me back to Mr W. He said, "There's nothing technically wrong inside you." He recommended I see a psychotherapist, but I just didn't want to know. I feel completely dead; I feel horrible about it. It would be worse if my husband were not so understanding. He is quite content to wait until I'm ready. It doesn't stop us being close. If anything, it's drawn us closer. I couldn't have a better husband really.'

When we talked to her, she was quite resigned. 'Now I've got to the stage where I don't think about it. If it's going to be all right, it will just happen. It's really depressing me, but hopefully it will come back.'

Now we turn to all the improvements reported. Our gynaecologist said that, although there wouldn't be any deterioration of sexual response, a woman shouldn't expect any improvement, but Jean's consultant put it a little more positively: 'We're rather giving you a present. We're taking away all the agonizing every month, and worry about whether you will get pregnant. We're going to save you chemist bills and so long as you can retain your ovaries, you'll not lose anything else.'

Unusually, Fiona's consultant mentioned orgasm. 'He said, "you will find you'll be able to have orgasm much more easily." And he was right. It's better and more pronounced. He didn't give a reason why it would be better, he just said it would be.'

It is easy to understand that a woman may well feel more pleasure from sexual activity when before the whole experience was dreadfully painful. The absence of pain allows a woman to relax more, to become more sexually aroused and therefore gain a lot more from the whole experience. 'Now he is able to penetrate fully. His body is against my body, and it wasn't before.' (*Fiona*)

'Once it was gone I knew I would be able to make love again. The important thing was to get rid of it so that we could return to our normal sex life again, which we did very quickly.' (*Celia*)

Jenny also found that the pain which had spoiled her pleasure of orgasm previously disappeared. Although it did take a little while before she could let go and trust that it wouldn't recur. Elaine reported 'only plus, the freedom of having no contraceptives.' Ellen, too, found it much easier having the freedom not to worry any more about contraception.

If a partner reports any improvement, this is again likely to be a consequence of the woman's increased capacity for relaxation and arousal in her own body. Everything will work more effectively because pain is no longer an inhibition.

It seems important that a woman and her partner be given adequate information beforehand. Our Staff Nurse felt it was very important to have the right advice, and cautioned against the danger of assuming that sex is only for the young: 'Every hysterectomy patient should be given the same opportunity to ask questions: it shouldn't just be taken for granted that because she's an old lady she wouldn't want to know this or that. Some women are still sexually active at seventy and you must be prepared for that as well.'

This Staff Nurse practised what she preached and established a relationship with her patients that made it possible for them to talk about the subject openly. She told us that she would frequently be waylaid between the shelves in the local supermarket by an ex-patient who would confidentially whisper, 'Tonight's the *night*, Sister,' with a meaningful nod and a wink!

11
Hysterectomy and Hormones

Most of us have a vague idea about hormones. But the precise nature of their operation in the body and their interaction with external stress remains elusive. This is true as much for the lay person as it is for the medical establishment who are still struggling to find scientific explanations for something they do not as yet fully understand.

Ever since the introduction of the contraceptive Pill, its rapid rise in popularity and subsequent decline, people have realized that when we interfere with the natural hormonal process we risk unpleasant side-effects. Consequently, many women have become sceptical about tampering with their natural hormonal balance.

In this chapter we look specifically at how hysterectomy can [illegible] this hormonal balance.

The Staff Nurse said that most women are aware that the ovaries are the source of their important hormones, and are therefore keen to hang on to them. 'It's the first thing they ask. They've got this thing about their ovaries. They know there's something there that keeps them young and beautiful.'

Jenny felt her ovaries were almost more important than her uterus. 'There was an element of doubt at the time, about what it might be necessary to remove and I was very keen to hang on to my ovaries. Much of my anxiety was due to the fact I didn't want to go through an early menopause. What would the drying out of my vagina do to my sex life; the ageing process, and the need for HRT? That was my worst fantasy.'

'I was particularly worried if I lost my ovaries what the effect would be on my whole body. Not just getting older, but having a very delicate hormone balance, thirty-three is a bad age to lose your ovaries. I suppose if you're older, you wouldn't notice it so much.' (*Jean*)

The significance of the ovaries meant that most of the women had discussed this with their consultant, though not all were anxious.

Elaine: 'They mentioned it but I wasn't bothered. It wasn't until afterwards that it dawned on me it might make a difference.'

'I was told that if my ovaries were healthy they would leave them in. But I didn't know when I woke up if I would have them or not.' (*Carole*) Both her ovaries were left intact.

'At the age of fifty-two, my ovaries would have started to shrivel up anyway, so I wouldn't have wanted them left in.' (*Sandra*) She didn't get the opportunity to discuss it beforehand but has since come to terms with it, even though she was worried at the beginning. 'I asked the registrar why I had to have my ovaries out. He said: "You don't want children do you?" I said: "But I don't want to get old too quickly." He said, "Oh well, these things do happen!"'

Celia had discussed it with her gynaecologist and had been given the information she requested. 'I was told they might have to remove my ovaries, so I knew it was a possibility.' (*Celia*) She had one ovary removed because of a cyst; the healthy one was retained.

Only two women in our group, Sandra aged fifty-two, and Sally aged twenty-nine, had both ovaries completely removed. Sally had one ovary removed two years prior to her hysterectomy but was still suffering very severe ovulation pain. In her pre-operative discussion she told her consultant she 'couldn't see the point of retaining the remaining ovary because that was the main problem.' She agreed to have the second ovary removed, and to be given hormone replacement therapy afterwards.

The menstrual clock

A hormone is a chemical substance produced in minute quantities by different glands in the body, in response to signals from the brain. The two hormones, oestrogen and progesterone, are produced in part of the ovary (the corpus luteum) each month during our menstrual cycle. The purpose of these hormones is to thicken the lining of the womb in preparation for the egg.

Studies of premenstrual tension show clearly that the presence or absence of these hormones can also affect our moods, physical co-ordination, body temperature, retention of fluid, skin texture and mental concentration.

Even after the womb and its lining are removed, the hormones continue to affect us in the same way. The pituitary gland in the brain, which signals the activation of the hormones, continues to do so even though our ability to conceive has been halted. The menstrual clock keeps ticking away, until the menopause, when it finally slows down and stops altogether.

After hysterectomy, women can still recognize the same symptoms which they already knew to be part of their menstrual cycle.

'I think my cycle is about six weeks. Not every month any more. I've not written it down, but I do get very bad backache on a regular basis – a pulling sensation round the back, but obviously no bleeding.' (*Margaret*)

Other women may experience breast tenderness at certain times; and others noticed swings in mood. 'Your hormones do take a battering. A year later, while I was busy on a course, I noticed over the three month period this feeling of disorientation; not being able to concentrate, and weepiness. It was twenty-eight days to the dot, on the button. My hormones had come back to a twenty-eight-day cycle. It was so obvious, it was marvellous.' (*Jean*)

Sally also experienced premenstrual symptoms: 'Angry outbursts, swollen breasts. My tummy bloats right out. There's nothing there, but it goes through the same process completely. I experience both the fluid retention and mental symptoms just the same.'

Ovaries are usually removed in the case of malignant disease. This applies if the ovaries are the original source of the disease, and where they are at risk of infection from elsewhere. Otherwise the general medical view is to retain the ovaries if possible as they serve such an important function.

However, some medical practitioners argue that it is a good idea to remove the ovaries because there is a 1 in 2000 chance that they might become malignant, and the female hormonal functions can be replaced with hormone replacement therapy.

'I think the balance of opinion now is that it's better to leave the ovaries and allow them to continue functioning. I think the patient is better off with normal hormones than supplementary hormones.' (*Gynae*)

Unfortunately, the medical profession seem generally to assume that once a woman has reached the time of her menopause, it is 'common sense' to take out the ovaries, because they don't have any further use. Although technically this may be true, and it may make the operation slightly easier to remove the ovaries rather than leave them in, it reinforces the unhappy tendency to view the human body as a mere collection of parts, rather than seeing it as something more whole and profound.

Hormone replacement therapy – HRT

The need for this therapy occurs when it is considered that a woman needs an artificial dose of chemicals contained in her hormones when the natural sources are inadequate.

HRT is used in the treatment of menopausal symptoms in women who are naturally going through their menopause, or women who experience an artificial menopause if their ovaries have been removed earlier in their lives.

If a woman's ovaries are removed long before her natural menopause is due, then she usually experiences very severe symptoms. On the other hand, if her ovaries are removed close to her menopause, the symptoms are not so severe.

If the uterus is removed but the ovaries conserved in a younger woman, her menopause will occur at the normal time in her life, unless the blood supply to the ovaries has been adversely affected at the time of the operation. A woman can only experience her menopause *once*.

Hormone replacement therapy is recommended to relieve unwanted symptoms of the menopause, whether this is the artificial or natural menopause. There are two main groups of hormones used in the treatment – oestrogens (most common), synthetic or natural; and progestogens which are often used in combination with the oestrogens.

Generally, oestrogens are effective in relieving psychological symptoms that are indirectly associated with oestrogen deficiency: insomnia as a result of night sweats, or loss of sexual drive as a result of painful intercourse. In addition, oestrogens can induce a feeling of well-being and energy in many women.

However, there is no evidence to suggest that HRT delays

ageing or prevents wrinkles or sagging breasts, although oestrogen therapy can improve the general appearance of the skin.

HRT involves administration of doses of natural or synthetic hormones (mainly oestrogen, sometimes progestogen) into a woman's body, in the form of a pill or an implant inserted just under the skin in the tummy, thigh or groin. In either form the dose is released at regular intervals as needed.

It all sounds pretty straightforward, as Sally thought: 'They told me I would need an implant once every six months. I thought, that sounds great, going back twice a year, that can't be bad. But it didn't work out that way.'

There isn't enough known about it, nor, as the Staff Nurse said, is there enough *said* about HRT. 'The patients don't know what to expect – they don't know if they'll get hot flushes, or start the menopause . . . women who have their ovaries removed should have more communication, and more frequent follow-ups, for the simple reason that if they haven't gone through the menopause, it can be quite a traumatic experience.'

Sally's experience certainly bears this out, and illustrates the difficulty of reliance on a form of medication that is, as yet, not thoroughly understood. Sally's hormone level was not tested before she was given the implant. This led to unforseen problems. She was expecting the implant to last six months, because that was what she had been told. In fact, the effect of the implant lasted just *seven weeks*.

At first 'I kept thinking I must be a bit of a freak, because it wasn't lasting as long as they said it would. I've only recently found out that this is quite common; it's due to your own metabolic rate. Being younger, we've all had the same problem, going six or seven weeks and then running out.' She always knew when she was running low because as the hormonal level dropped, her mood changed drastically. 'When my hormone implant ran down I was at my lowest. I couldn't cope with anything else and that made me depressed. I got very weepy at the slightest thing. And I lost a lot of weight. Luckily, my husband noticed it. He wouldn't tell me before because he thought I'd get worse. But I say to him now, "please tell me", because he can see the signs as it's approaching, and I know then I'm not imagining it.'

The first time the implant ran out prematurely, Sally returned to the hospital for more and was told the reason it hadn't lasted was because 'after the operation they reckon your body uses it up quicker, but then they said it would slow down. But it happened again.'

A further difficulty was that Sally had to travel to London because she couldn't get her HRT implant locally. This meant there was always a delay between her recognizing that another implant was due and being able to obtain one.

'By the time I was due to have the third implant, I had to wait five weeks in between doses. During that time I went down and down and down. When you have the next dose it takes that much longer to get to where you were in the first place. It's a vicious circle. Each time they gave me a different dosage which they haven't got quite right yet. At first they gave me oestrogen only. They normally start you on that, to help with the sweats. But I had a low energy level. Then they gave me testosterone to go with it; as it ran out so quickly they gave me a double dose, which must have upset me because I was very hot and bright red. The HRT never lasted more than seven weeks.'

Sally kept a detailed diary of what happened to her, and wrote to her local gynaecologist who recommended she try tablets. 'I thought, I'm game for anything, so long as they make me feel better.' She was prescribed a low dose oestrogen tablet, and synthetic progesterone for three months. Despite premenstrual symptoms recurring, she persevered and went back to see her local gynaecologist when she ran out of tablets.

Unfortunately, Sally never managed to see the original gynaecologist again. She was referred to a much less sympathetic assistant who threw Sally's carefully prepared diary notes into the waste paper bin, commenting all she could do was 'give me a repeat prescription of the same tablets. She as good as told me I would always have to rely on something or other, and put up with the consequences or go without. I was so shocked, I didn't say anything. Coming home I burst into tears.'

After this episode she went back to her own GP who arranged for her to return for further treatment to the teaching hospital in London she had attended before. When we interviewed Sally she had just received notification of her appointment – it was *seven months* away. As she said herself: 'What I'm supposed to do for these seven months in between I don't know.' Meanwhile, Sally has to live with premenstrual symptoms. 'Will it always be like this? Will I always have PMT? Eventually it will go away, but no one knows when. In one person it might go away in a matter of months, in another, a matter of years. I didn't realize that.'

She also has to depend on a flawed system of drug manufacture and distribution. 'The existing system for obtaining hormone treatment means they can't overlap the doses, it always has to drop first which really shouldn't happen. They told me I would have to have HRT for the next 15 years – that's a long time to have to cope with ups and downs. You don't mind it taking a little time to get right, but you want to stick to some kind of level eventually. And now because of an administrative hiccup, I've got to wait seven months for my next appointment. Fortunately, I got some tablets for the interim which I stretch to tide me over I hope, but it's not ideal. I shall keep persisting until I get a better answer.'

Understandably, Sally has strong views about HRT and is anxious to help other women considering the same treatment. 'As we are all individuals, it is very difficult to gauge the right dose of hormones. I think if anyone is told they will need HRT after the operation, they should request a hormone test *before* having the treatment, whether an implant or pills. You must know what your hormone level should be normally and ensure that you are carefully monitored so that your hormone level is maintained.'

Confronted with the removal of her ovaries as a *fait accompli*, Sandra's experience was different. She went to see her gynaecologist who suggested it would be a good thing to go on HRT. She felt very positive about it: 'HRT is my idea of retaining some youth. I don't see why you have to age just because you have to, when there's a means to prevent it. I started off on my HRT and I still have it. I tell my GP what I want and we have a laugh about it, because he says, "You know more about it than I do."' (*Sandra*)

Sandra found that the hormone replacement therapy she took in tablet form alleviated unwanted menopausal symptoms: 'After my hysterectomy I got hot flushes and used to wake up at three o'clock every morning. That has gradually disappeared and the flushes have stopped.'

Sandra seemed to thrive on HRT and, in fact, her problems only arose when, at her GP's request, she started to reduce the dosage. 'I got it down to half a dose per day and tried to tail it off rather than stop abruptly. But I started getting very touchy and miserable again without them. I'd snap back at people, and got very weepy, so now I've gone back on to the full dose.' At the time of our interview, Sandra told us that she and her GP were in strong disagreement: 'He is now getting to the stage when he wants me to stop. But I think I ought to carry on. I'm determined to stay on HRT.'

One other woman in our group had some experience of HRT for a short while. Margaret was very depressed and visited her GP nineteen months following the operation because she was uncertain whether her emotional problems were as a result of hysterectomy or other things going on in her life. She was given HRT for three months: 'I was trying to understand why I felt like I did, which was a bit horrible. I didn't want to speak to anyone and I withdrew into myself. My hair stopped growing, and my nails as well. I noticed my hair because it grows quickly normally and I didn't have it cut for three months. I didn't have to shave under my arms for three months either. When I stopped taking the tablets, my hair grew again, and my nails.'

HRT after Hysterectomy – What the Experts Recommend

'Some known side-effects of HRT are fluid retention, headaches and obesity. More dangerous side-effects include deep vein thrombosis, or pulmonary embolism [blood clot in the lung].' (*Gynae*)

Of course, there are conditions under which it may be unwise to use oestrogen replacement therapy. This is why each woman would benefit from being able to discuss her difficulties with a sympathetic clinician or doctor.

It is astonishing how little of the ovary is required for our normal hormone level to be maintained naturally. Even though Fiona only had half an ovary retained after her hysterectomy, it functioned effectively enough for her to avoid HRT completely. 'They said that if I needed HRT after the operation I could have it. They told me the the symptoms I would have if I needed it – hot flushes, feelings of agitation, general tiredness. I had to wait a period of three months before they decided. I didn't have any of the symptoms, so I didn't have HRT.'

It is virtually impossible to predict which dose of hormone therapy would be suitable for an individual woman, or how long she will be required to continue treatment. It is important if not essential, that a woman be assessed *before* treatment begins, to ascertain the normal hormone level. Her weight and blood-pressure must be measured and her breasts and pelvis carefully examined. It is also important that this assessment be repeated at regular intervals during treatment.

Once treatment is underway, it is worth discontinuing therapy from time to time, in order to discover whether you still require to continue with hormone replacement artificially.

Our gynaecologist was very much in favour of HRT as long as there was no history of illness or disease that could be aggravated by the treatment. Although not specifically related to hysterectomy, he felt that, without HRT, there was no other satisfactory way to avoid severe symptoms that some women suffer in their natural menopause.

He added that women were likely to come up against prejudice about HRT in their own GPs. 'I am amazed to encounter it – the tremendous prejudice within the profession. It starts with the medical students, even before they've done any gynaecology.' (*Gynae*)

This is how he described a common experience in his teaching role: 'Every time I take a group of medical students I say to them, "Now imagine you are doing a GP surgery for the first time. The receptionist says this is an easy one, she just wants another prescription for her HRT. What would you do?" Most of them will have all her clothes off, thoroughly examine her, take her blood-pressure, do a smear and then warn her of the risks she's running and try and get her off it.

'Their view is that you shouldn't be on drugs for a long time and anyway, there is a risk of cancer. Then I say, "What risk? The risk of cancer is not clearly documented and it doesn't occur in patients who have HRT three weeks out of four with progesterone supplements. Where do you get this idea from?" They don't know. I've spoken to the Professor of Therapeutics, he can't explain it either. We just don't know where they get it from but they are all quite keen to stop HRT.

'I say to them, "Well, if I'm the GP and I hear you've stopped this woman, who might be a widow running a small business, has to attend board meetings, needs all her drive and enthusiasm, and doesn't want to be caught in a little black dress with a big sweat mark, I'll sack you." They get even more angry. I say, "You must never stop treatment that another doctor has started unless you've got a very good reason for doing so." Prejudice against HRT starts very early on. I think it's prejudice against women being kept young.' (*Gynae*)

So, although HRT can be highly effective, it is important to be aware of the existence of this kind of prejudice. It is also important, before embarking on this treatment to ensure you are adequately assessed and continuously monitored. And finally, to remember that no one yet has all the answers about hormones and exactly how they work. 'We do not know all there is to know about the metabolism of oestrogen. There are so many variations between women. Some do not suffer severely when the ovaries stop functioning and some do. There is no scientific explanation for this.' (*Gynae*)

'It's still experimental and they don't know how each woman will respond: we are still guinea-pigs.' (*Sally*)

Afterword:
'Will it Make a New Woman of Me?'

'No one should assume that everyone has the same experience. There are some generalities, but the fact that it's difficult for one woman shouldn't make us all think we are going to have a difficult time; likewise things that are easy for some might not be easy for others.' (*Jenny*) The variety of descriptions expressed by the women in this book certainly confirms Jenny's statement.

If thought and care are taken in the first place, it does seem that hysterectomy can make a positive difference to some women's lives, even though it may take time: 'Now I think hysterectomy is wonderful. Four years later, I do feel much better.' (*Angela*)

Obviously, there are practical advantages as a result of having no more bleeding and pain. 'I just feel so much better and it still continues to improve – I can't believe it.' (Ellen) This increased energy and zest for life was mentioned by several of those women who had spent so long feeling utterly drained.

But apart from the more predictable benefits, we were interested to hear two women describe an unexpected but profound change in their self-esteem, which reinforces the mystery element of the uterus in terms of self image:

'I feel very much less vulnerable. I seemed always to be apologizing for things before. If it was raining, I'd say, "Good morning, I'm sorry it's raining." I wouldn't dream of doing that now. I was always trying to please people before and felt guilty about things which were not really my fault. Now I don't. People must take me as they find me and if they don't like what they see, I don't mind. They don't have to look. I can now go for things I want and not feel that I have to give an explanation and consider everybody else before I do something I want to do. It's been a very marked change and a very good change as far as I'm concerned.' (*Fiona*)

Carole's comments were very similar: 'The hysterectomy has given me a security. I can't explain it. It's not because I can't have any more children, because I was sterilized before I had the operation. It's really weird but I don't mind what people think of me now. If I'm fat, I'm fat. Now when people make comments about my weight, I say, "So what! I'm fat and happy!" I used to worry about what my parents thought about what happened in my family; I was frightened to tell them things that had happened. Now I've opened up and I'm more outspoken with them. I say, "It's my family so it doesn't matter what you think." Before, I was still their little girl. But now, I feel I've found myself.'

Further Information

Judy Vaughan
WIRRAL HYSTERECTOMY SUPPORT GROUP
Rivendell
Warren Way
Lower Heswall
Wirral
Merseyside L60 9HJ

(This organization can put women in touch with counsellors around the country who have experienced hysterectomy. They are willing to share their experience and support you throughout your hospital stay by 'phone, letter or, if near enough, personal contact. Please send a stamped addressed envelope for more information.)

HYSTERECTOMY SELF HELP
11 Henryson Road
Brockley
London SE4 1HL

(This is another counselling organization started by Ann Webb, a Health Visitor. Support groups are held at the above address on a two-monthly basis and include an informal exchange of views and experiences on hysterectomy.)

Gynaecological advice and menopause clinics are available at the Departments of Obstetrics and Gynaecology at the following hospitals throughout the United Kingdom. A referral note from your doctor is required before an appointment can be made.

LONDON – NHS

Chelsea Hospital for Women
Dovehouse Street
London SW3 6LT
01-352 6446

King's College Hospital
Denmark Hill
London SE5 9RS
01-274 6222

Hospital for Women
(Soho Hospital – part of
Middlesex Hospital Group)
Soho Square
London W1V 6JB
01-580 7928

St Thomas' Hospital
London SE1 7EH
01-928 9292

Royal Free Hospital
Pond Street
London NW3 2Q9
01-794 0500

Samaritan Hospital for Women
Marylebone Road
London NW1 5YE
01-402 4211

St George's Hospital
Blackshaw Road
Tooting
London SW17
01-672 1255

Dulwich Hospital
East Dulwich Grove
London SE21 3PT
01-693 3377

ENGLAND – NHS

Women's Hospital
Professional Unit
Queen Elizabeth Medical Centre
Edgbaston, Birmingham B15 2TG
021 472 1377

Birmingham & Midland Hospital for Women
Showall Green Lane
Birmingham 11
021 772 1101

Royal Sussex Hospital
Brighton, Sussex
0273 66611

Women's Hospital
Leeds
0532 453905

Dryburn Hospital
Durham
0385 64911

The Lady Chichester Hospital
New Church Street
Hove, Sussex
0273 778 383

Beckenham Hospital
379 Croydon Road
Beckenham
Kent
01-650 0125

City Hospital
Hucknall Road
Nottingham
0602 608111

The General Infirmary
MRC Mineral Metabolism Unit
Leeds
0532 32799

Women's Hospital
Gynaecological Clinic
Catherine Street
Liverpool
051 709 5461

Wythenshawe Hospital
Southmoor Road
Manchester 22
061 998 7070

Manchester General Hospital
Crumpsall
Manchester M8 6RB
061 740 1444

Mexborough Montagu Hospital
Adwick Road
Mexborough
South Yorkshire
070 988 5171

Newcastle General Hospital
Westgate Road
Newcastle upon Tyne NE4 6BE
0632 38811

George Eliot Hospital
College Street
Nuneaton
Warwickshire
0682 384201

Peterborough & District Hospital
Thorpe Road
Peterborough
0733 67451

Jessop Hospital
University Department
Sheffield
0742 25291

Royal Hallamshire Hospital
Glossop Road
Sheffield S10 2JF
0742 26484

Stafford General Infirmary
Stafford
0735 58251

Ashford Hospital
Staines
Middlesex
07842 51188

Stepping Hill Hospital
Stockport
Cheshire
061 483 1010

The John Radcliffe Hospital
Oxford
0865 64711

SCOTLAND – NHS

Aberdeen University
Foresthill
Aberdeen
0244 234423

Glasgow Western Infirmary
Dunbarton Road
Glasgow G11
041 339 8822

Royal Infirmary
39 Chalmers Street
Edinburgh EH3 9ER
(Newington) 061 667 1011

Glasgow Royal Infirmary
Castle Street
Glasgow G4 0SF
041 552 3535

Stobhill Hospital
Balornock Road
Glasgow G21
041 558 0111

WALES – this clinic is not NHS but is free to patients

Simbec Research Centre
Merthyr Tydfil
0685 2324/2533

NORTHERN IRELAND – NHS

Samaritan Hospital
Lisburn Road
Belfast
0232 41316

EIRE – NHS

Coombe Hospital
Dublin 8
0001 757561

Other Useful Addresses

ELIZABETH GARRETT
ANDERSON HOSPITAL (EGA)
144 Euston Road
London NW1
01-387 2501

FAMILY PLANNING
ASSOCIATION (FPA)
27-35 Mortimer Street
London W1N 7RJ
01-636 7866

(FAMILY PLANNING
INFORMATION SERVICE
at same address – free publications list)

INSTITUTE OF PSYCHO-
SEXUAL MEDICINE
11 Chandos Street
London W1
01-580 1043

ENDOMETRIOSIS SOCIETY
65 Holmdene Avenue
London SE14 9LD
01-737 4764

MARIE STOPES CLINIC
Well Woman Centre
108 Whitfield Street
London WC1P 6BE
01-388 0662 *and* 01-388 2585

ROYAL LONDON
HOMOEOPATHIC HOSPITAL
Great Ormond Street
London W1
01-837 3091
(centre for alternative medicine)

WOMEN'S NATIONAL
CANCER CONTROL
CAMPAIGN (WNCCC)
1 South Audley Street
London W1Y 5DG
01-499 7532/4

WOMEN'S HEALTH INFORMATION CENTRE
52 Featherstone Street
London EC1

(National information and resource centre for women's health issues. Run by women working in the health field as health workers, teachers, writers and researchers. They work with and act as a resource for women in health groups, community groups, trade unions and other women's groups.)

WOMEN'S HEALTH CONCERN
17 Earls Terrace
London W8 6LP

(Provides information and advice to all those who seek help with health problems. WHC concentrates mainly on gynaecological conditions and its medical experts try to help doctors to look at women's health problems seriously and to treat them with appropriate medical or other suitable treatment, whether symptoms are caused by physical or emotional illness.)

Booklist

Hysterectomy, Wendy Savage (Hamlyn Pocket Health Guides, 1982).
Hysterectomy, Elliot Philipp (Family Doctor Booklet, British Medical Association).
Hysterectomy, Dennerstein, Wood, Burrows (Oxford University Press, 1982).
Whose Body Is It? Carolyn Faulder (Virago Press, 1985).

Glossary of Terms

Adenomyosis: Condition in which cells like those in the endometrium, are found embedded in the muscular wall of the uterus.
Adhesion: Fibrous tissue which often forms after an operation; adhesions can bind organs together causing pain and discomfort. They may also interfere with the proper function of those organs.
Amenorrhoea: Absence of menstrual flow.
Anaemia: Low level of the red pigment carrying oxygen (haemoglobin) in the blood.
Anticoagulant drug: A substance that prevents clots forming in the blood vessels.
Anti-prostaglandins: Drugs which can be successful in preventing menstrual pain, and excessive menstrual bleeding.

Biopsy: Removal of small amount of tissue for microscopic examination.
Bladder: Balloon-like organ which stores urine.
Bowel: Section of alimentary canal below stomach, intestine, gut.

Calcified fibroid: Sometimes called a wombstone, an old fibroid which hardens as deposits of calcium salts build up over the years.
Cancer: Malignant growth of cells.
Catheter: Narrow tube inserted into the bladder in order to drain it.
Cervix: The lower part or neck of the uterus where it joins the vagina.
Corpus luteum: Yellow mass formed in the ovary after the egg has been released.
Curettage: See D and C.
Cyst: A swelling filled with fluid.

D and C: Stands for dilatation and curettage: dilatation means the cervix is stretched open, and curettage means the removal of the lining of the uterus. Often known as a 'scrape'.
DVT: Deep veinous thrombosis; clots which form in the deep veins of the legs and obstruct blood circulation.

Dysfunctional uterine bleeding (DUB): Excessive bleeding and pain caused by heavy irregular periods.
Dysmenorrhoea: Painful periods.

Embolism: The transfer of a clot in the vein from one part of the body to another causing an obstruction, e.g., pulmonary embolism – an obstruction in one of the arteries in the lungs.
Endometriosis: The growth of cells normally present in the lining of the uterus, in other parts of the pelvis.
Endometrium: Mucous membrane lining of the uterus which grows each month to be shed during menstruation if pregnancy has not occurred.

Fallopian tube: Tube down which the egg (ovum) travels to the uterus.
Fibroid: Lumps of fibrous tissue which grow in the muscle of the uterus. They are not a form of cancer.
Fibromyomata: The full name for fibroids.
Follicle: Very small sac or gland containing mucous substances.

Gonadotrophins: Hormones produced by the pituitary glands which act on the gonads (ovaries in women/testes in men).

Haemastasis: When the bleeding stops.
Haematoma: A clot caused by blood which has escaped from its proper vessel into the tissues, following injury.
Hormone: A chemical substance produced in minute quantities in one part of the body and carried to an associated organ by the blood stream where it greatly influences the activity of that organ.
Hormone replacement therapy: HRT is the artificial administration of hormones in tablet or implant form, to replace those no longer naturally produced by the ovary.
Hot flush (or flash): Sensation of warmth which 'flashes' over the body, especially face and neck.
Hysterectomy: Removal of the uterus (for details of different types see pages 72 and 76-8).

Laparoscopy: A minor operation using a surgical instrument like a telescope (laparoscope) to examine the organs in the pelvis, through a small abdominal incision.
Ligaments: A tough band of fibrous tissue connecting bones or supporting organs within the abdomen.

Menopause: When the menstruation cycle ceases in a woman's life.
Menorrhagia: Heavy prolonged bleeding.
Menses: Menstruation.
Menstrual cycle: The number of days from one menstruation to the next, during which regular hormonal changes occur.

Menstruation: The cyclic discharge of blood from the non-pregnant uterus. Usually occurs at approximately four week intervals.
Micturition: Passing of urine.
Myomectomy: Surgical repair of the uterus to remove fibroids.

Oestrogen: One of the female hormones produced in the ovaries.
Oopherectomy: Surgical removal of the ovary.
Orgasm: Peak of sexual excitement.
Ovarian hormones: Oestrogen and progesterone which produce a ripe egg each month.
Ovaries: The organs situated in the pelvis above the uterus on both sides which produce eggs and hormones.
Ovulation: The time during each month when one or two ova (eggs) are released from the ovaries.

Peritoneum: Thin membrane lining the abdominal walls and the outside of the uterus.
Pituitary gland: Gland at the base of the brain which produces many hormones governing the process of the menstrual cycle.
Polyp: A smooth rounded knot of tissue growing from the endometrium or cervix.
Progesterone: A female hormone produced by the corpus luteum, which works in harmony with oestrogen.
Prolapse: The displacement of any organ from its normal position, as in prolapsed womb.

Salpingo-oopherectomy: Removal of the Fallopian tube and ovary.
Sarcoma: Cancerous-like growth in muscle or bone.
Speculum: A metal or plastic instrument used to see inside parts of the body such as the vagina.

Thrombosis: Formation of blood clot within the heart or a blood vessel.

Ultrasound (scan): Very high frequency sound waves used to transmit a picture of internal organs on a TV screen.
Ureter: The tube carrying urine from the kidney to the bladder.
Uterus: Womb

Vagina: A tubular canal leading from outside the body to the uterus.
Vault: Upper part of the vagina into which the cervix protrudes.

Index